Adventures In Home Birthing

Adventures In Home Birthing

Making Babies And Having Them At Home

RahLeeCoh Ishakarah

aka Doctor Daddy

To order additional copies of this book, contact:
Xlibris Corporation
1-888-795-4274
www.Xlibris.com
Orders@Xlibris.com
67102

DEDICATION

TO THE MEMORY
OF MY MOTHER

WHOSE TOUCH BROUGHT
BARREN CLAY POTS
TO FLOURISH
WHOSE LOVE BROUGHT
TRUTHFUL DEVOTION
FROM MY FATHER

WHOSE LOINS BIRTHED
STRONG MEN-CHILDREN
WHOM SHE NOURISHED &
GUIDED TO MANHOOD

WHOSE BREATH GAVE LIFE
TO A JUNGLE OF GREENS &
VINES & LEAVES
AND
WHOSE MEMORY EVOKES VISIONS OF TRANSPARENT
LIME GREEN AFRICAN CONTINENTS . . . . PROJECTING IN A ME
ROOTED IN DOWN HOME SWEETNESS, SO SINCERE,
WARM AND GENUINE, WITH ONLY "FOR REAL"
FEELINGS FOR ALL . . . .
THANK YOU MAMA
RahLeeCoh

PREFACE

If your wife attempts to turn a friend into a live "shish kabob" using a ninja sword, . . . or, if she strips and threatens to run out into the highway, to dance with on coming traffic, or if she helps you to bring your 100 yard dash time down using a butcher's knife as incentive, while, at the same time . . . has an increase in trips to the urinal, along with developing strange appetites for weird combinations of food at odd times of the night; and, if she also has sickness and nausea every morning, . . . you can be pretty sure that the chances are great that you have really scored this time, and she is "going to have your basketball!"

As advocates of home birthing, my wife and I offer this humble record of our birthing experiences, which includes the steps we follow to bring our children into this world. In support of such advocacy and self reliance, we've found that having a strong "working" faith in God is the most important prerequisite to getting ready and being prepared for the demanding responsibility of being a spiritual attendant assisting your wife, as she allows God's natural forces to guide the birth of "you-all's" new baby. *(In case you have not figured it out yet, this "work" is written from a male perspective, wherein the expectant father is charged with the responsibility of managing and orchestrating the birth of his own child. He must also accept the responsibility of caring for the health and protecting the well being of both mother and child.)* This means, in turn, that the "attending father" must acquire and possess certain knowledge and skills, including:

1. An understanding of the basic principles of Alternative Healing Systems;
2. Knowledge of Holistic Health Care and sources in the Bible for strength and confidence in the use of traditional healing methods;
3. Research and study of literature, such as "Spiritual Midwifery," and case Histories of pregnancy fitness and birthing stories;
4. Some understanding of applicable Allopathic theory, method and practice.

In addition to the foregoing wisdom and information, we found it very beneficial and comforting (particularly to ease "Mother-To-Be's" initial fears) to discuss our plans with an Allopathic Practitioner who was sympathetic to natural birthing methods. We were lucky and blessed that this doctor was herself a mother, who had delivered her own children at home, not only naturally, but also, all by herself.

We also conferred with Mid wives, nurses (male and female), and Naturopathic Practitioners, all of whom provided valuable insight that prepared us for our first home birth. That first successful birthing allowed us to gain experience and confidence enough to bring forth the rest of our ten children without further assistance or consultation.

Thus, we herein offer our reader benefit of our accumulated successes and expertise, in hopes that it will clarify and simplify the notion of home birthing, and eliminate the fear and uncover the mystery, to help those parents who wish to embark on a similar course, by offering them the "road map" my wife and I had to discover from empirical research, counsel, trial, and an overpowering desire for a true picture of natural birth.

At any rate, we pray that those who read the following account and stories (some of which have been embellished, and with some name changes) will be entertained, enlightened and amused by the humorous, yet serious recollections of our "Adventures In Home Birthing," which were guided by our love for one another, and our faith in God.

TABLE OF CONTENTS

INTRODUCTION

To prepare the reader for the information, assertions, and stories about the home child birth blessings God gave my wife and me, we begin with a brief overview of the very factors that led to our success: 1) the importance of father's role as "Mid-husband;" 2) the recognition and understanding of, as well as the appropriate response to what we regard as the first signs of pregnancy; 3) necessity for trust in the power of God for the source of strength to handle birthing responsibilities, and faith in God for direction; 4) birthing room preparation, methods and purpose of controlling birthing environment; 5) getting prepared to assist baby into this world, as well as being ready to handle problems that may arise; 6) being sensitive to "Mama-to-be's" emotional outbursts, and other signs that clinch our belief that "Mama" is pregnant; and, 7) acting on the foregoing belief by immediately starting to get "Mama" ready for the birth.

Throughout our discussion of the above factors, we use colorful and interesting stories of relevant birth experiences to illustrate the important ideas and points unique to the birthing procedure God allowed us to uncover and follow.

Though we do not wish to get too formal in our presentation, we do want the reader to seriously consider the underlying holistic medical wisdom upon which our actions are based, on the basis of its viable merits. So, we do include thought provoking information and controversial concepts from legitimate sources and authorities in the field. And, though we consider the act of childbirth as a spiritual phenomenon, we, nevertheless, attempt to be scientific in our methodology, particularly as it relates to our systematic approach to observations and data collection surrounding our immediate pregnancy and birthing preparations. However, even though we include these organized, yet "aborted" records, we also include the reasons we abandoned such an ambitious goal hidden in the sad story lines of a possible miscarriage.

But, before we get started on our exciting adventure, we must also include notations on the theoretical justifications for our choice of actions (only in the interest of scientific validity, since our faith precludes such need), as well as the health principles upon which our decisions are based-the foundation of what we view as spiritual directives.

A final note before we get into the "fruit" of our "journey," concerns the frame of mind that is conducive to undertaking this awesome task. It is essential for Dad to exhibit a sure and confident attitude, which stems from the belief that God will protect and oversee the birthing. The expectant Mom must feel this trust and certainty, to help allay the milieu of fears that confront "both" prospective parents' minds. This is important because mother's mental state affects the way her body functions, and in turn the manner in which baby grows inside her womb.

FIRST SIGNS OF PREGNANCY

It all begins for me when I observe certain changes in my wife's behavior, and conditions of her body that signal to me that she is pregnant. The following list of changes set my "Mid-husband's" instincts into motion (these indicators do not include the feeling that I got on two occasions that actually signaled a state of pregnancy-namely, the feeling that "I just launched the big one," and it would hit the target!): 1) First, there is the "missed menstrual cycle;" 2) Then, there is an onslaught of "morning sickness" and persistent "day nausea;" 3) Next, there is an increase in urination; 4) Then, there is an increase in appetite, including cravings for weird combinations of food (junk food gorging) at odd times of the late night; and, 5) Finally, the clincher for me comes with the advent of that inevitable cloud burst of bizarre responses to what she says I have or have not done or said.

As I mentioned earlier, this last sign is pretty convincing evidence for me, that sometimes takes the form of "naked ninja mama to be," in need of assurance that some younger, or maybe sexy woman is not getting, or not going to get daddy's love, affection, attention and or time.

The presence of all the above signs is positive proof for me; I know that it is time for me to start working with Mother's dietary and spiritual needs. However, earlier in our "baby making" experience, we also relied upon "over the counter" pregnancy tests, as well as other so-called modern medical means and methods for confirmation. But, as we explain later, we grew spiritually to the point of avoiding such methods in favor of faith in God and reliance upon divine revelation, not only for positive proof of pregnancy, but also for direction in the management of the whole process.

As an experienced dad who has assisted mom in bringing forth new life, those signs not only indicate to me the existence of a fragile state of mind in need of a constant show of love, but also an imbalance of nutrients, as the developing embryo actually takes its nutrition from mother's body. It is at this point that I become more sensitive to my wife's feelings, and I make a conscious attempt to be more understanding. This means, instead of falling prey to senseless arguments (that I can't win anyway), I gather my self-control and give in to her wishes. I grab hold of her and kiss her eyes and mouth, rubbing and soothing and calming her. I was more successful at mustering such discipline during the earlier pregnancies. Now, with the pressure of the demanding needs from all our other children, my drained state of mind is a little slower at moving from conscious recognition and reasoning to administering appropriate solutions, and taking restorative actions.

It is also at this point that I see the need to implement a dietary regimen that includes pregnancy vitamin supplementation, increased amounts of fresh vegetables and fruit, as well as increased amounts of fresh squeezed fruit and vegetable juices, especially spinach, carrot, and apple/celery combinations. This, of course, is in addition to our family's regular vegetarian diet, which we have not maintained firmly of late, yet not to the point of violating our "no meat" policy.

Mama's dietary regimen includes drinking a lot of herb tea, the most important of which for Mama Akua (Mamaku) is Squaw Vine and Red Raspberry. (As Mamaku drinks these two herb teas religiously when she is pregnant, we order them in bulk.)

Mamaku declares that this diet, particularly the two herbs just mentioned, is responsible for the fact that her pregnancies with our last six children (the first three of our nine were conceived during her previous marriage) were much less painful. She goes on to assert that her labor time is a lot less, and less mucus is produced, the babies are cleaner, and the problem of clogged respiratory system and obscured eyes is practically eliminated.

JUSTIFICATION FOR FATHER'S ROLE AS SPIRITUAL BIRTHING ATTENDANT

As "father to be" is most likely the closest person to "mother to be" and the developing baby, he should be able to feel the changes, and subsequent needs of his growing family. Since he is also charged with the responsibility of providing for the care of this family, it is my sincere belief that every man who impregnates a woman should also accept the challenge of participating in the birthing process. I also believe that said man should take control of the situation and manage his own procreative development. By taking such initiative, the prospective father sets into motion certain positive forces that can only help to strengthen the bond between his family, building confidence, trust, and greater love within this "holy trinity."

I sincerely believe that this act of procreative management is more spiritual and Godly than scientific and technical. Thus, it is my contention that, by conducting the reproductive process accordingly, we may solve many of today's societal problems, especially those related to human interaction, more specifically those involving strained relations between mother and father, and also between parent and child. Further, I feel that the father's involvement in the birthing process creates several positive side effects. First, it increases dad's sensitivity to mom's needs and develops a sense of mutual worth and importance. Secondly, it increases the chances of creating a situation that generates more love and greater understanding, while allowing for more tolerance of individual differences and male/female peculiarities. This may mean longevity for the union because of the closeness caused by the sharing involved in such an intimate and caring experience. Such a total commitment by "father to be" could also be the catalyst needed to restore the family unit to its position as the cornerstone of our American society. And, finally, by acting as spiritual attendant and conducting his own baby's birth, he saves the family thousands of dollars in medical fees; there is an inevitable boost to self-esteem for all involved; and, both parents will have demonstrated courage and heroism, as they have vanquished real and imaginary demons and foes-the biggest of which is fear.

As we intimate in Chapter 5, fear is an enormous negative motivating factor that "father to be" must overcome to ensure the safety of his mate and unborn child. This potentially disruptive negative force can be controlled to a great extent by the steps taken to "order the room selected for the birthing" (It is more manageable when you "stay on the battlefield-in this case, the birthing arena-with trust in God.").

BIRTHING ROOM CONDITIONS

The knowledge and experience my wife and I have gained from delivering our babies at home lead us to believe that one of the most important determinants of a successful home birth lies in the atmosphere and conditions that exist in the room chosen for the birthing. In our case, it is our bedroom. We are careful to ensure that this room contains a loving mood, a healing spirit, and the sweet feeling of peace that comes from the comfort of a fresh, cleaned and ordered space.

I must admit that most of this work is done by Mamaku, usually during the "eleventh hour" (except in the birth of our baby girl, Namibiyah, whose delivery stage arrived just minutes after Mamaku began painting frantically on the wall where our unfinished baby bed would rest). It is at this stage of the birth process that "mother" receives a superhuman burst of strength and house cleaning energy. Mamaku fondly refers to this phenomenon as "nesting." This intense state of enormous energy build-up supplies the labor power needed to disinfect beds, rooms, and furniture, and, organize, clean, sort and arrange affairs to accommodate the coming "down time." So, when I witness this stage of development, it serves as a wake-up call, I become sobered to the fact that it won't be long before the top of that wrinkled little head will be peeping up through that blessed pee hole.

It is also at this time that I assist Mamaku by handling some of the other methods we use to create the proper atmosphere and generate the correct frame of mind needed for a smooth delivery (if that's possible). We've found it helpful to establish a spiritual mood by burning incense (preferably frankincense and myrrh). We also create a peaceful and calm environment by playing soft music, such as chanting sounds or songs from the "easy listening" radio station. I also create a warm, cozy and serene feeling by replacing the overhead light with a bulb that glows with a blue hue.

In addition, I brew us a pot of healing herb tea. The tea selection is either the pregnancy "blend" that Mamaku created, or a calming tea such as, catnip or valerian root.

Also, there are several things that we do to sustain a loving atmosphere. For one, we do a lot of touching and caressing. During these tender moments, I massage "Mamaku's vaginal area," rubbing in olive oil to reduce the possibility of tearing the "taint." I do this, while "sweet talking" to her, using flowery words to reassure her, and to compliment her regarding her faith, her courage, and her beauty. I thank her for having trust in me, and I applaud her "working faith" in God, including her conviction when it comes to being fruitful and multiplying. I am careful to let her know that I love and appreciate all our children; making certain that she understands that we all need her, as she is irreplaceable. This acclamation and show of love may not be enough reassurance later when the pains get more severe. At these times, I've had to hold on tight and ask for forgiveness for my many faults and a sin or two. She has been known to confess at such times also, as we cling to one another for strength and support. The idea here is that "mother to be" needs to be free of mental constraints and worries as much as possible, to ensure that her body functions are not restricted or negatively affected by avoidable stress.

Before we get ahead of ourselves and begin describing the actual birth, it is safe to say that a birth room full of warm, loving, ordered, sanitized and spiritual vibrations is essential to a successful birthing. This atmosphere, including the soft lights, gentile and soothing sounds, and, healing tastes and smells provide a proper background and setting for the birth of our children. Miraculously enough, we achieved all these conditions about thirty minutes prior to "count down and blast-out," for delivery of our last two children.

We were also blessed with a peaceful serenity resulting from the fact that all our other children fell asleep at the same time.

In order to be totally prepared with the right birthing room conditions, it is also necessary for all tools, materials, and supplies to be ready and available in a handy location next to the bed. (Don't be surprised-like I was during our son Jolanti's birthing, if you can't remember where you put the clamps, blades and sterilized sheets and towels, as an overwhelming presence causes your mind to go blank. Your wife, as did mine, may remember "in the nick of time, "and calmly guide you to the night table and dresser drawer where everything is waiting; or, she may suddenly remember that she packed all the tools away in the traveling bag, because we just returned from a trip and were prepared to deliver, regardless of where we may have found ourselves at that moment.) At this point of readiness, we also keep the Bible, "Male Practice" by Robert S. Mendelsohn, "Positive Pregnancy Fitness," and "Spiritual Mid-wifery located in a handy place for quick reference, because we often get the urge to review certain sections of these books just prior to delivery, or immediately thereafter. Don't be surprised also, if you are "led" to an important section, where you obtain valuable information that you will need only moments later, when you arrive at a "hairy" situation requiring specific "know-how."

As you can imagine, gaining all the knowledge needed for this job requires a total commitment to health improvement, and wellness, which means including study time in your lifestyle that is devoted to exploring the Healing Arts, as well as other sources of information related to contemporary and traditional medical wisdom and practices. You may want to gain first hand knowledge of the efficacy of such methods by "practicing on thy self." Don't despair though, "fellas;" don't let this task seem too monumental. A good thing to remember is that trust and faith in God makes all things possible, including the delivery of your own child, by you, in the comfort and sanctity of your own home.

FAITH IN GOD'S POWER AND ALTERNATIVE MEDICAL KNOWLEDGE

We cannot stress it enough that the first condition that must exist in the minds of "mom to be" and "dad to be" which sets the stage for a safe home childbirth is a strong belief and faith in God. This includes an unyielding trust held by the expectant father that God oversees, guides and protects his course of naturopathic action. For the expectant mother, this trust supports her faith that her unborn child's "attending" father receives the divine strength, skill and knowledge needed to "see" them through the birthing safely.

Of course, my wife's decision to allow me the chance to deliver our children was also influenced by the fact that she knew that I have over twenty years experience as a student of the healing arts. Nevertheless, it took quite a bit of coaxing for me to convince her to try the natural birth method. The two things that finally convinced her to give in to my wishes were one: the sobering stories told by Dr. Robert S. Mendelsohn regarding some horrible consequences to mother and baby when certain modern medical procedures and equipment are used for diagnosis, monitoring and delivery, and two: the painful state that certain prenatal procedures she received from a local women's clinic left her in, after each visit-a bloody, hobbling condition that I was forced to correct, using massage, herbs and oil.

As you can see, the knowledge of Alternative Medical systems, and Holistic Health Care is almost an indispensable prerequisite to taking on the awesome responsibilities associated with giving birth to your babies at home. For that reason, anyone wishing to achieve the kind of success my wife and I experienced would do well to obtain knowledge and understanding in Herbology, Vegetarianism, Yoga, Reflexology and Massage Therapy.

If you can accomplish all these feats in advance of the "twelfth hour," you are in good shape and prepared for the adventure of "having" your baby at home. Yet, as we suggest throughout, it is possible even without this background, if your faith in God is strong enough.

CHAPTER 1

FATHER'S ROLE AS SPIRITUAL BIRTHING ATTENDANT

The movie industry loves to paint a picture of the expectant father as a man so nervous that he "freezes" and even faints at the sight of blood from his mates womb. He is portrayed as utterly useless when his baby begins to push into this world.

It is true that at the instant my babies' wrinkled heads pop up into view-usually after much coaxing, blowing, sweet talking, panting and crying out-that wet, "grayish pink wonder" awes with such mesmerizing force that the feeling of catatonic immobility overwhelms my senses. So, it is possible for one to become too numb to take action or make any movements. However, such languishing luxury can only be entertained for a "nanosecond." The urgent reality that my wife and unborn child need me, and depend upon my level headed command of the situation forces me to quickly overcome the "swooning" feeling and take control of the situation. I get control after much praying to God for a sure hand and an alert mind; it is a sustained prayer that continues as I perform the rapidly unfolding tasks.

This brings to mind circumstances surrounding my last baby's (Namibiyah's) birth, which occurred on August 14th, 1995. That event was enough to let me know that you cannot rely totally on past birthing experiences to dictate your every move. It reminded me that I must stay close to God for strength, protection, problem solving, and insightful decision-making.

This birth did not go according to schedule; our previously laid plans went out the window, and, my wife and I were not as prepared as we have been for past births. I was not in denial of the closeness of the moment of truth, yet I didn't believe it was as close as it turned out to be. I based my presumptions on several facts. One, . . . we were not ready yet! My wife had not completed her usual "nesting" chores, with the corresponding surge of motivating superhuman energy, which usually lets me know that it is time to get everything in order. In fact, on the morning of the due date, she insisted that I take her to Jackson State University. So, even though she continuously told me she was in labor. I was fooled by the fact that she had given me false alarms all that week. Those previous false contractions lulled me into thinking that she must not be that close (she didn't tell me until recently that she really knew it was time; she also knew that the important business matters she had to take care of could not wait until she recuperated).

Looking back on that day, I remember that it began routinely enough; Mamaku took her usual early morning stroll; on this morning, however, she stopped by the phone booth on the corner of Capitol and Denver Streets. She called our oldest daughter-Nika. She asked Nika to drive by our house on the way to work, and allow her to borrow the car to finish some last minute business. Mamaku dropped Nika off at work and returned home for the rest of us.

So, . . . there we were, early that morning, all of the children piled into that little blue Neon, me driving, and Mamaku more pregnant than I suspected.

While the children and I enjoyed the scenery of Jackson's urban University (JSU), Mamaku took care of business that took quite awhile. During that time, we met two enthusiastic exchange students from South Africa. They were fascinated with us, as we were with them; we had Dred Locks in common, which my wife found remarkable given the things we heard about Apartheid in their country. Little did we know, the name of their hometown-Namibia-would prove to be so very significant later on that day.

Meanwhile, after Mamaku came down from the JSU Towers, where student records are kept, she insisted that I take her downtown to the Social Security Office.

At the Social Security Office, the children and I escorted Mamaku to the elevator, but we did not stay for two reasons. First of all, since all three of our vehicles were broken down and in need of repair, and I was behind on my own business too, I took that opportunity to use the car to conduct some business of my own. More importantly though, security around the Federal Building was nervous and jumpy, due to the recent bombing of that same facility in Oklahoma. So, waiting outside (or inside) was not such a comfortable idea.

When I returned a little while later, Mamaku was sitting on the steps of the building, and a nervous Social Security Administrator, who was smoking a cigarette, stood watch over her. She was obviously relieved to see me. (I discovered later that this sweet lady had entered the hall from her office door to find Mamaku in a Zen position, meditating and panting, on the floor in front of the elevator. So, we see that the nervousness was not due to threat of bomb, but threat of delivery. Yet, I still didn't have a clue.)

As soon as we arrived home, an unexpected guest pulled up into the driveway behind us. It was Q—a friend of the family, who had attended a Holistic Health Care seminar hosted by my wife and I, in our home, for Jackson State and Tougaloo College students. "Q" needed me to assist him with my auto mechanic skills. After I determined that his battery needed charging, which explained why he was having difficulty starting his car,

I hooked my battery charger up to his battery. I did this in a hurry, while informing Q that my wife was in labor, yet, also telling him that I felt we had a couple of hours before delivery. Since his wife would also be giving birth to their first child soon, I suggested that he could come in when the battery was charged, and watch, and perhaps even assist me in the delivery. (I really wished that he would take advantage of this opportunity because he and his wife had intimated to me that they wanted me to deliver their baby. But, I tried, unsuccessfully, it seems, to let him know my feelings on the subject, which is that each and every man who impregnates a woman, should, with blessings from God and the expectant mom, help deliver his own. So, I attempted to let him know that I would be available to assist him with his child's delivery, but, as I am not a licensed doctor, I could not put myself in the position of being liable. I pleaded my case, stating: "Q, I feel that this should become a "man thing", wherein we as expectant fathers assume responsibility for the delivery of our own babies."

As fate would have it, Q did not come in to witness the birthing; he missed an experience of a lifetime, that may have inspired him to conduct his own (which he did not; he allowed a midwife to handle it). It became quite apparent that he was not coming, after much time passed, and I needed help, but was unable to leave the birthing room. I discovered months later that he had simply placed the battery charger inside the screen door when he was finished charging his battery, and then drove to East St.Louis.

Oh, . . . but, lets back up a bit, . . . to when I left Q, and finally went into the house. It was then that I became aware that ALL HEAVEN HAD BROKEN LOOSE.

After closing the front door behind me, and making sure that I didn't lock it, so that Q could enter, I heard a commotion. As I started down the hall, oblivious to shiny hardwood floors, an entry gallery of fine art (my own creations), and, walls and base boards that were waiting for their usual disinfecting before delivery, I could hear my wife; her mouth was in rapid perpetual motion, as she "blessed me out." In a high pitched voice, she lamented and wailed that she did not want to have the baby, and that I would not be there when the baby came out. She moaned that my friends were more important than she. Then, . . . she yelled that she couldn't take the pain!

When I reached the bathroom, she was climbing out of the bathtub. Her appearance startled and puzzled me at the same time. She had drops and smears of white paint everywhere, and the sink was full of paint water and a partially cleaned paint roller. As she stepped onto the cool vinyl floor, she continued drying off with a big warm fluffy towel that she had just taken from the dryer. When she paused her verbal assault long enough to lift her head, she screamed at the sight of me! She exclaimed: "It's too painful . . .

this early (so she thought), . . . I got too long to go before the baby comes. That's when the pain will be much greater." She caught her breath, as she toweled her hair, and went off, again: "I can't take it, I can't take it."

Quietly, I assisted her to the bedroom, "splitting myself in two," so I could stay with her, yet at the same time, clean up the mess of a half finished paint job, which, to my dismay and surprise greeted me in the bedroom. She had half finished the two walls where our baby bed and dresser were to go, whenever I finished restoring them. She accomplished this unfinished bit of "nesting" in the short while I was outside with Q.

She was off and running now. She continued wailing at me in a higher gear now: "You don't love me anymore. You have treated me very badly throughout this entire pregnancy."

Of course I didn't agree with this position, but I kept quiet, as I hurriedly attacked eleventh hour preparations in the twelfth hour. I did this as swiftly and as humbly as possible, absorbing verbal blows, and muffling mental responses to disputable charges. Unlike times of late, I was able to choke back my argumentative replies to a ceaseless barrage of vocal accusations.

Luckily, the children went to sleep about a half hour before all this excitement began, just as mysteriously as they had done so in the previous two births. However, as I attempted to juggle paint brushes, rolling pan, buckets and other painting paraphernalia, along with a pot of hot water for herb tea, clean sheets, sanitized towels (sterilized by baking in the oven wrapped in brown paper), and clean up tools, I became acutely aware of the fact that I needed my oldest daughter's assistance. In this mad frenzy, I also realized that I couldn't remember where I put the sterilized clamps and blades. I thought: "Oh yeah, there're in the night table! . . . Right? Wrong!" My mind raced frantically. "How would I cut that cord and clamp it?!."

To top this off, instead of my usually calm expectant wife-mother, who had control of all elements of the birth situation, this time, unsteadied by recent rough relations between our selves, Mamaku was uncertain, fearful, and, her faith in me seemed shaken.

I had to calm her down, though, some how; consequently, I began to rap to her. In a soft, sweet whisper, I reassured her, as I picked her up from her Zen position at the foot of the bed. Accepting my turn at labor, I scooted her from the spot where we dropped in bed. I did so by placing my hands under her arm pits, and "inching" my way to the head of the bed. All during this backbreaking work, I repeatedly and rapidly encouraged her, proclaiming: "You can do it Mama . . , you've done it many times before. You are beautiful and strong, and God is watching over us. I'm not going anywhere, not now or ever."

I said these words as she began lamenting out a non-believing response: "Naw, you gonna' leave me; you won't be here when the baby comes."

I had to bring her out of her hysterical state of hyper-sensitivity, so I quickly responded by repeating the same sweet words that I just "ran on her," adding: "I'm sorry Mamaku. If I hurt you, it was not my intention. I never want to disappoint you; I always want to love you, and our family." I continued in soft desperation: "and, . . . Honey, we need you . . . , don't give up. You are strong, and you can handle it. God gives us our crosses to bear, and He gives us strength enough to carry them."

I said this as I thought to myself: "How in the hell am I going to get to that kitchen! How in the world am I going to do all the things I need to do without leaving and alarming Mamaku. If I move from her presence for just one second, she will be convinced she was right, and that would send her deeper into hysteria."

Just then, even before I could get that thought completely out of my mind, as I simultaneously massaged her belly, and puss, and the spot that can tear, smoothing these areas gently with olive oil, a powerful eruption caused Mamaku's "public place" (as Grady from Red Foxx's old show used to say and call it) to suddenly swell. Her vagina quickly grew like a volcano, peaking to reveal the wrinkled top of a little head.

I thought: "Lord, her water bag must've broken while she was in the bath tub, and she didn't realize it."

It was clear now, that even though Mamaku was screaming "bloody murder," sure that she was in the early stages of labor where the pain should be less intense and more bearable than in the later stages, we were actually there at the instant of birth.

According to my calculations, which I based on the time frame established with our previous birth experiences, she was really ahead of schedule. In fact, I felt that this was the quickest delivery time yet.

Lo and behold, . . . before I knew it, out popped a cute little head.

Inside my head, my mind's ear was nearly numbed by a deafening affirmation I yelled to myself: "Hey, . . . that face looks like mine!"

I was so proud of my "touch down run," I could have danced happily in the end zone. However, I didn't have even one second to celebrate, because, immediately I was shaken by the next sight. The umbilical cord was wrapped around the baby's neck! Once again, I was startled by "such a sight," like that which occurred during the birth of our youngest son at that time-Rah-Imhotep.

Yet, this time, it was an even more frightening sight! I gasped out a few barely audible words, as I pretended to be calm, in order to disguise and conceal my alarm from my wife: "the cord is wrapped around the baby's neck." (Actually, I think I said "his neck," because I believed this was a boy. I based this belief on the fact the baby had strong features that resembled mine so very

21

closely. I was not sure of the baby's sex because we choose to wait until God reveals this fact to us. We do this for the purpose of adhering to Natural Laws, and to avoid the harm that may come from submitting to the use of monitoring devices and x-ray machines. According to Dr. Robert S. Mendelsohn, in "Male Practice," these modern procedures and equipment pose a potential threat and may be dangerous to the unborn baby's health and life!)

Surveying the situation quickly, I could see that, unlike 'Hotep's cord, this umbilical cord was wrapped tightly around the baby's neck. I tried in vain to get my fingers underneath the cord. My wife sensed the danger. She accommodated my unspoken wishes instinctively by controlling her pushes. She pushed only hard enough to allow just the baby's shoulder to emerge from her womb.

My knees were knocking and my heart was pounding so loudly that I was sure my wife could hear. So, I began praying silently, asking God for forgiveness for any and all of my sins, . . . "our" sins. I continued by asking God to keep my hands as steady as stone, because I didn't want my wife and my "borning" baby to feel the fear that gripped my knees, my legs, and my heart. A great deal of this fear was due to the fact, as I previously noted, that for the first time in all our births, my wife let me know that she was afraid. This meant that I could not draw upon her strength and faith in me for energy and certainty.

But Holy Hallelujah! . . . . My prayer was immediately answered! My wife began to sweet talk back to me! Imagine that; she actually asked me to forgive her! And, . . . she told me that she loved me; this gave me renewed energy to continue on with the cord.

Funny thing was, though, despite the intensity of the moment, I was really prepared for this particular wrap of the umbilical cord, because only hours earlier, as I brushed up on delivery stories in the wonderful little book, "Spiritual Mid-wifery," I read a section which dealt with such an emergency. However, written words are one thing, but living the reality is a thousand others. At any rate, the book didn't prepare me for the sight of my suffocating baby, whose face turned a cold blue, and whose lips turned a scary purple.

Even so, it seemed a commonsensical matter to just grab the baby's hand, and thread her arm through the cord. But, to my dismay, my baby's hand fought mine fiercely, slipping and ducking with uncannily adept moves. Nevertheless, I caught her hand and slipped it, just in the nick of time, carefully and quickly, through the cord, which had become slack only after the shoulders emerged.

Then, after quickly "slooping" the cord over the baby's head, before the next wave of contractions came to push her all the way out, I finally saw that the baby was in fact a woman child.

Hold on, though, . . . my worries were not yet over. After I lifted my baby girl out safely, the tension-which was relieved by the safe delivery, immediately began to build again; because I could not locate the clamps and sterilized blades! I was alarmed for Mama Akua's safety.

Again, my mind began to race frantically. Suddenly, Mamaku interrupted the brewing frenzy; she remembered that she carried those items in her purse all day, because she secretly felt that the moment of delivery was nearer than she led me to believe.

I could now sigh with relief and remember that in all this time, I had been unable to get to the kitchen. But now, after I lay the baby on Mamaku's warm thigh, took the clamps out of their sterile packet, clamped the cord in two places-about an inch apart, and about an inch and a half from the baby's belly-I took the blade from its sterile container, and cut the cord, I was finally able to get into the kitchen to prepare Pennyroyal herb tea.

Mamaku drank the tea, and we waited for the placenta to deliver, as she squatted.

A half hour later, the placenta slowly eased down into my waiting hands, which I held cupped underneath Mamaku. Relieved, I carried the "mountain oyster" looking tissue to the back yard, after carefully allowing it to gently separate from the walls inside the womb. I located an appropriate spot, and buried the placenta, but not before finding a plastic bag and a shovel. Now, I was satisfied, proud and happy.

Upon returning to the "scene of the birthing," I commenced to clean up soiled, bloody and wet sheets, and towels. I was happy that God had showered us with blessings-a healthy and safe Mama and child. I was so elated as I performed my chores that I thought about the seven dwarfs in "Snow White," when they sang: "Just'a whistle while you work." (I even whistled the tune they did—whistle, whistle, whistle whistle) As I did so, a song "welled" up inside my released spirit, forcing itself out from my lower belly.

In a low guttural chime, near Shabba Ranks type raggae pounding sound, the following lyrics flowed from my "Chi," with an undeniable and timely revelation:

> "I'm a Mississippi Dred Lock Bah Bah, with a Bop-a-T-Bop"
> "I put D Baby In D Mama, and I take 'em out too;
> The Good Lord showed me just a what to do"
> "I'm a Mississippi Dred Lock Bah Bah with a Bop-a-T-Bop"
> "The pretty babies keep a comin', and they just wont stop . . .
> . . . they "jes" wont stop"
> (I repeated this stanza over and over and over, until it
> stuck in my mind.)

23

But, before I could finish singing my melodic expressions of joy, my children-who had now awakened with excited exclamations of wonderment-joined me in my song of merriment. Somehow, their creative imaginations reached a simultaneous and brilliant accord. They added their own instinctive lyrical expressions of happiness and gaiety in a thrilling harmonious background accompaniment:

"Doctor Daddy"
"Doctor Daddy"
"Doctor Daddy"

As their cute little voices and dancing bodies chimed in synchronized unison, pelting out the above phrase, over and over again, a grin spread across my face and illuminated my soul.

That was a wonderful little side trip, but lets get back to the Father's Role as Spiritual Birthing Attendant, and conclude this chapter.

If the birthing story we just reminisced about seemed a bit "hairy," we hope that it does not discourage any potential mid-husbands from accepting this challenge. Actually, out of all our deliveries, we've only had one other birthing that was really alarming. All things considered, our deliveries, especially the first-which occurred in the back seat of a cab, went swiftly. Further, there were no long bouts with intense and unbearable pain (if you let me tell it), like that experienced by most mothers; and, the babies we birthed at home were clean, unclogged with mucus, alert and looking up with bright, open eyes—ready for mother's nursing (all our yunguns but Namibiyah were ready for ninny immediately).

The most important point to remember here is that the expectant Dad will achieve the best results, and obtain the greatest assurance of success when he calls upon God for direction. Of course, as you may well imagine, it helps to be prepared with knowledge gained from study of appropriate literature, along with consulting professionals in the field, including nurses, mid-wives, physicians, and traditional healers, or practitioners of Alternative Medical Systems. In my opinion, your chances for success are increased, if you "know the herbs of the field." In addition, I attribute our own home childbirth success to the fact that my wife and I did not hesitate to seek the aid of our friends to obtain needed materials and supplies, as well as advice for relief from anxiety and fear, and to gain confidence and self assurance. It is also important that you remember to have the house, your business, and the birthing room clean, sanitized and in order, with necessary implements stored in a handy place, well in advance of the so called "due date."

Oh, . . . by the way, we left our last little story so quickly that I forgot to mention that Mamaku and our baby girl-whom we named Namibiyah (remember the students from Namibia?) Lilli-Lee Raspberry Verderosa Ishakarah, had to spend about two weeks sleeping in the children's room. They had to wait until I finished decorating our bedroom. It was well worth the wait! "Doctor Daddy" was pleased with his handy work, which included cream lavender walls and shiny metallic gold trim. This was accented by the baby's matching glossy white dresser and baby bed, which sat on a coordinating tiny blue Oriental rug. This area was sectioned off from the rest of the room to appear as if it were a separate room sharing the same freshly varnished hard wood floor. We were happy to get back into our new room, thankful for the opportunity to enjoy a nice new environment, complete with ceiling graphics. It was perfect, not only for recuperation purposes, nursing and "loving," but also for entertaining friends and family, who were curious to see our new baby.

As you can see, all came out well, but this example illustrates the point that the perspective parents need to be ready and careful not to depend totally on past experiences for direction. They must be prepared, open to potential scenarios, and flexible, with available options.

For me this birth was affirmation of our faith, and conviction that childbirth is a spiritual phenomenon, governed by the will of God. Consequently, any deviation or interference with this divine plan runs the risk of causing complications, or unnatural and indefensible results!

CHAPTER 2

GETTING MOTHER READY

Throughout all of my wife's pregnancies, she follows a few important procedures to the point of making them her birthing rituals. She does this to maintain wellness, increase her strength, and ensure good health for our unborn child. Not only does she begin a strict dietary regimen (this diet includes herbs, vitamin and live food therapy) that allows for the unborn child's nutritional needs, as well as her own, she also assumes a Pregnancy Fitness Program that contains scheduled activities-including exercise, prayer and meditation sessions, and a lot of walking.

But before we get too far ahead of our selves, lets back up to the point when I decide that it is time to start Getting Mother Ready. As I mentioned earlier, despite all other signs that indicate the possibility of pregnancy, I become convinced that Mamaku is pregnant when she has a profound and even bizarre emotional out burst. Then, the first thing I do is to take steps to protect her fragile mental state-which includes satisfying her need to be pampered, and indulge her unusual (diet busting) junk food cravings.

I didn't always possess this pregnancy assessment knowledge, or the ability to make the correct response to apparent "psychological-imbalancement" problems-which were probably due to vitamin mineral loss to the baby. There was a time when I did not have the wisdom of a considerate and sensitive mate, thinking and weighing my words before speaking. I can still remember the incident that awoke me to this reality of human (female) nature; it allowed me to develop the proper attitude and the option of selecting an appropriate course of action.

My revelation came during the pregnancy of our daughter Rahkua, who is now 8 years old. At the outset, Mamaku knew, but I didn't have the foggiest idea that she was pregnant. I was not yet sensitive to the signs that reveal the state of impregnation; the following recount reveals the manner in which I became forever knowledgeable of those signs and their importance in determining when to start Getting Mother Ready:

At that time, we maintained separate living quarters; she had her own home (which she lost as result of the repercussions from her unlawful termination (unlawful, according to Judge Fred Banks), which we discuss briefly later), and I had my own home as well. The incident occurred during

26

one of my visits to her house. She had reached that emotional state where they (wives and girl friends) bring up everything bad and negative that ever happened between the two of you (not to mention also, all those things that happened with all the men of their past). This argument put too much stress and pressure on my normally understanding, sweet and kind nature (smile). So, when she asked me if I were ever going to marry her, my frustrated and badgered mind led me to reply: "How can I marry you on this starving artist's income . . . , and besides, I didn't know that you could curse me out like this." Oh yeah, I was on a roll now, why not air all my pent up grievances, so I continued throwing my usual understanding attitude out of the window, I added: " . . . and, I can see now, how a man can be pushed to the point of brutally beating one of you women (before the reader jumps to the wrong conclusion, I have never hit my wife)!"

I had been pushed too far this time, though, and that was what she needed to hear; . . . . right? . . . Wrong!

I should have been thinking, "Oh Lord, what the hell did I say that for!" . . . Because, I was not, in my wildest dream, prepared for what came next.

She quickly responded, as if reading from a prepared script, by saying "Oh, and who the hell am I; . . . what am I, your little "throwaway" or something? What, . . . I'm not good enough for you, hungh?!"

Sparks were flying from her eyes, and lightening bolts shot from her erected "Dred Locks." I started to back up a little, . . . eyeing the front door, as my "wife-to-be"-whose face was now a grimace of red fire-began ripping off her clothes.

When she turned and bolted for the kitchen, since I had never witnessed anything like that before, I figured it was time for me to ease on out the front door, while I was still able.

Before I could reach the end of the front porch, our oldest daughter's screams caused me to turn around in time to glimpse her clinging to her mother's arms-which were attached to hands that wielded a great big black butcher's knife!

I immediately leaped off the porch, and grabbed one of the big logs I had just cut for the fireplace. I wheeled around in time to swat that flying butcher's knife out of the air. I did so, just before it could reach me. I caught the gleaming blade that reflected the cool colors of the clear Mississippi night air; it stuck straight and taught, held by the permissive fibers of the freshly ax hewn southern pine.

Completely naked, and dragging daughter behind her, Mamaku was moving fast and screaming. She was screaming something about "not being loved" and "always at fault." She raced toward St. Charles Street. Since her

27

house was very close to the street-about 30 feet away-I had to move in haste to catch her. Mysteriously enough, St. Charles Street-which was usually busy at this time of evening-was empty and lonely; so too was the surrounding neighborhood. There was a strange and deserted feeling that permeated the atmosphere, and was masked by an early evening darkness, which was filled with clear cool air.

"Thank goodness, no one is out to witness this madness," I thought, as I chased Mamaku down, and caught her before she reached the end of the drive way. I quickly wrapped her up in my arms and carried her back to the porch, where daughter stood wailing, and flailing her arms and body. She screamed in a frightened voice: "I'm going to call my Daddy!" (She cried these words, even though an ugly divorce stood between her blood parents, long before I arrived on the scene.) I reassured her, as I naively informed her that her mother was o.k. "She just mistakenly assumed that I don't love her," I said, while restraining Mamaku in an arm lock that contained her body in a loving manner.

How innocently naïve was that of me, . . . to believe what I had just said, and then slip away to freedom, after gently and carefully releasing Mamaku.

It took me about five minutes to walk home, anxious to get to the sanctity of my own bachelor pad.

It was not your typical single man's house and abode-you know the ones that look like they need mom, or the attention of maid service. It was my sanctuary: a shiny cherry/mahogany hard wood display temple for my art. It housed my creations, my many and varied schools of original artistic thought and expression, countless number of styles and media, including exact likeness pastel portraits, wood carvings, drawings, abstract paintings, framed prints, aluminum spaceships, and much more. There, in my Studio home, I was protected, and fulfilled by the realized promise of peace, solitude, and positive interaction, with no contrary feedback, nor retorts of disagreement.

But before I could reach the safety of my private sanctuary, I was startled out of my single-minded quest! A fast approaching vehicle seemed to be headed toward me. As I neared my driveway, it became quite clear that the car, now speeding, was intent on running me down.

It happened so fast, that, there was only one thing to do. I did an O.J. Simpson; you know, where in the T.V. commercial he jumped over rental cars, while running to catch a flight. Well, I was taking flight all right, and during that leap, I took a look into the windshield of the phantom vehicle. I was startled again. It was my "wife-to-be!" It had all happened so fast that I hadn't recognized her car. But, I knew those eyes.

As I landed from my flight over danger, I don't remember needing feet to carry me over the distance between the driveway, my front lawn, or the high cement steps to my front porch, where I reached the front entry door. However, I do remember two luminous red dots, penetrating the opaque blackness inside the car; they followed me, angrily piercing my being with a murderous looking "eye-ray."

Peeping through the sheer baby blue curtains that adorned the pane in my front door, I thought: "What in the hell have I gotten myself into this time?"

Then, when the "phantom-car-never-more" finally abandoned its vigilant street corner perch, squealing off in a mad rush for destinations unknown, leaving rubber and chaos in the upset dusty air of its wake, it dawned on me. I was no longer blindly naive. I exclaimed out loud: "Aw man, she's pregnant!"

So, men, if you can recognize those signs before tire tracks rearrange your chest hairs, I pray that you will appease and calm your mate down with a sensitive and understanding touch. I hope that you will lighten her heavy psychological and physical burden with kisses and kind words. For, what profit a man to win an argument, and his woman to lose control of all reason? (In the reader's mind's ear, I wish the preceding passage heard as if delivered by a voice that sounds like a combination of that of my Grandfather-Rev. M. H. Herron, who loved to quote the inferred biblical scripture, which deals with the fisherman of men's souls-and, Aretha Franklin's father-Rev. C. L. Franklin, who was our family's pastor in Detroit, when I was a youth still living in my mother and father's house. I want the reader to hear that question asked in a voice that sounds like one with a down-home southern tremble, harmonized with a sophisticated northern, big city refrain and moan.)

I wish someone had warned or advised me of those possible changes that a pregnant woman may go through. But, then, its "kinda" relieving, and afterwards, isn't it fun to recall?

Seriously, though, at this time-once I have witnessed the "far out" behavior-when I am convinced that Mamaku is pregnant, I feel it necessary to take certain steps to keep her in a state of serenity. I surround her with as much love and happiness as possible. I steer clear of conversations and issues that I know will set her off. I take every opportunity to let her know how much I love her, and how much we need her. I also say to her as often as I can: "You are beautiful, and I'm happy and blessed that God put us together." I make a special effort, as well, to remind her that she is the answer to my prayers, wherein I asked God for her and for our children.

When Mamaku gets pregnant, I take steps to circumvent thoughts she may have that doubt her self worth, and her sexual desirability. This is necessary because our society places a premium on the slim model image, while at the same time, a negative stigma is placed on a woman who fruitfully multiplies. So, I let my wife know that she is still, and always sexy to me. I convince her that she doesn't have to feel insecure about her size and shape, and that I cleave only for her. In addition, I make sure that she knows that my love for her is more spiritual than physical, and goes deeper than skin or penetration.

Another important note on considerations to keep in mind while you get mother ready for the birth has to do with our belief that mother transmits thoughts, feelings, and emotions to the unborn child. For this reason, my goal is to keep Mamaku happy, satisfied, and as calm as my frail human psyche allows. So, when Mamaku gets those candy bar cravings at 3:00 A.M., even though our health teachings warn us to avoid all such "foods," I, nevertheless, faithfully trudge out into the cool pre-dawn moonlit darkness, to the nearest convenience store to obtain the "sweet" needed to satiate her "jones"-usually a Baby Ruth or a Snickers. Though I am aware of the potential danger posed by a dose of concentrated sugars (and toxin) to her system, I figure that emotional disturbance caused by denial, and mental turmoil the result of self-righteous preaching would be more harmful than limited indulgence. Usually these cravings follow one of our late night reading sessions, which-during these periods of pregnancy awareness-we devote to reading (out loud and to one another) everything we can surrounding the topic of childbirth and natural delivery at home.

We admit that our foregoing discussion of how I get Mamaku ready for birthing concentrated primarily on mental preparation, yet her physical preparation is equally, if not more important. She usually takes charge of this responsibility herself, which includes a scheduled agenda of exercise-which we obtain guidelines for executing, from "Pregnancy Fitness," a book designed for the purpose of keeping mother fit throughout the pregnancy. The exercises include workouts involving my participation, as well as those using chairs, pillows and the floor for feats like pulling, stretching, and lifting. I generally conclude these sessions with an olive oil massage and over all rub down of her entire body. Then there are the daily walks, which entail journeys through our neighborhood, usually early morning and late evening, and which sometimes includes the whole family. During these walks, I most always accompany Mamaku, but she has been known to go alone, and even with a pregnant companion or two, as well. Though we have fun and greet a lot of people on these walks, (they have even generated a style of art creation I invented from recycling and reconstituting the aluminum cans we collected for a period), the idea is to strengthen the body, with special attention given to the areas that will get the greatest stress during delivery.

Suffice it to say that my considerations are many when I decide that Mamaku is pregnant, this includes her dietary needs-which will be discussed later when we examine her food in-take regimen. My job is to ensure that she is prepared both mentally and physically for the task of childbirth, by making sure she has the essential vitamin and mineral in-take needed for her body to perform correctly, while providing the developing baby with what it needs to develop properly. We get these nutrients from commercial vitamins and minerals, healing herbs, fresh fruit and vegetables (and their juices), nuts, grains and spring water. The bottom line is that we want to make sure that Mamaku's body functions at an optimum level of efficiency, and her mind is happy with the idea of bringing forth new life for our family.

CHAPTER 3

BIRTH ROOM PREPARATIONS AND READINESS

My wife and I were most ready and best prepared for the birthing of our last son—Rah-Imhotep. We arranged and ordered the birthing room, and other important matters, and, got everything under control, well in advance of this blessed child's entry into this world. (Rah-Imhotep lives up to his namesake. In fact, on many occasions, he, without having been informed or requested, comes up to us and places his hands on an unannounced painful area of our body and commences to rub the pain away in such a loving and unbelievable manner.)

With God's blessing, and the help of a few good friends, we were able to take care of all the details related to the birth of this son. We finished the domestic chores, arranged financial affairs, scheduled business obligations favorably, and completed all other tasks, at least two weeks prior to Mamaku's due date. However, this experience taught us that players from this world do not possess the ultimate power over the baby's birthing destiny. (This clinched our belief that only God has this power, particularly when it comes to natural birth.) We also became aware of the fact that, even though you may have it all together, and think that you are ready, you can still be caught off guard, and have to solve unanticipated problems.

Two weeks prior to the due date (Mamaku has developed uncanny accuracy in predicting her own due date), we received two clamps and blades in sterile packets, from a friend of ours, who is a nurse (Sadly enough, we have not seen this friend in a long time-perhaps because of the following incident that occurred the last time we saw her, which we feel obliged to share. It happened when she stopped by to see the little baby, for whom she provided invaluable delivery accessories).

Shiela was a friend of our family, because her husband Mitchell and I go way back; he used to be my next-door neighbor and auto mechanic compatriot. As she stood on our front steps talking to my wife and me, I sat on the porch, at my easel, drawing and painting a portrait using pastels and air brushed acrylic on canvas.

Suddenly, a well-dressed young Blackman—one you wouldn't think to be a culprit-strolled up to Shiela's car, just as easily and confidently as you please. Shiela had left the car running; it purred helplessly in my driveway, down hill of our position at the top of our high front steps, some thirty feet away.

Then, the young man, who appeared to be well mannered, dressed in a walking suit, wearing clean white sneakers, with a clean cut demeanor, tipped his hat to us. Without any resistance from the vulnerable vehicle, he boldly and calmly opened the door. And, without threat or malice, "just as pretty as you please," he said: "Thanks for the car!"

Our disbelief turned into astonishment, as he quickly swung himself under the steering wheel, and just as quickly and smoothly, backed the car straight out onto an empty West Capitol Street.

Before the little unlikely crook could turn, straighten up and pull off, "sister-girl" bounded the steps in a single leap, reaching the street almost instantly. She was intent on preventing her car from leaving. However, "brother-man" was serious, and did not hesitate to nearly run her over, save for the fact that she avoided the front bumper. He was getting away, leaving Shiela jumping up and down, pleading with me to stop him.

I was far ahead of her though. I had already leaped over the 16-foot metal sign, which I salvaged from my last sign job. It was an antique Coca Cola Sign, and I used it to block the entrance to our front porch, in an effort to keep our children from running out into the usually busy Capitol Street, which leads through the heart of the city, and ends at the Old Capitol Building, two blocks from the Governor's Mansion.

In two bounds, I too landed in the driveway, only farther up, near the side of the house; where our cute little, newly acquired Dodge Ram Mini-van lay in wait for such an opportunity to shine. My efforts were stalled a bit, though, as "fumbleitis" prevented me from getting my key into the ignition switch.

After what seemed like a thousand years passed, I finally managed to get started. I quickly backed up (without taking the emergency brakes off, which I didn't remember until this adventure was over). I stopped long enough to pick up Shiela. She was hysterical! I pulled off in time to see her car disappear over the distant horizon, where the Amazing Grace Church sits, left of the blind curve at the top of the winding hill on Capitol Street.

I punched the gas on our sweet little "family-vehicle." It responded immediately, and we flew in perfect time, because I had just given it a tune-up.

Over the hill, and through the light at the zoo, we sped. We zipped past the Fire Station, unable to catch sight of the stealing away vehicle yet. We wondered if he might have turned down one of the side streets; but, since he could have only turned left, it was a safe bet to take quick glances up the streets, as we sped by them.

When we finally reached the bend in Capitol Street that unwinds in view of Ellis Avenue, I spotted her car. It was speeding through the light. (The traffic must have been heavy enough to block his get away.) We too made that light. We also sped through the next light, which was turning red. We lost sight of Sharon's car until we passed that light at the old abandoned Barefield Hardware building. We were in luck though, because we moved swiftly enough for me to catch a glimpse of the car turning left onto Alabama Street.

I floored that Dodge Ram Mini-van, and cut in front of some fast approaching automobiles. I cornered Alabama with a wide arch. As I rounded that street, I did so in time to see the red luminous parking lights illuminate the fast approaching darkness of dusk. As her car pulled into a driveway, thick shrubs, which grew all the way out to do the street, concealed it, but not the red glow reflecting through the shrubs like Christmas tree lights. That quick hiding place might have evaded our searching pursuit, were it not for the hazy red glow on the dark green sculpted leaves, which lasted only long enough for the half slick young man to stop the car.

The trick did not work, and the chase was over. I eased right up behind him, just as pretty as I pleased.

Shiela had been jumping up and down in her seat throughout this entire real life chase scene, yelling: "Go faster RahLeeCoh, catch him. Don't let him get away with my new car (some kind of a pretty little foreign "job")." She yelled these words over and over again, until she had begun to sound like the "Amen Corner," when they coax a down home Southern Baptist Preacher to his squalling climax.

Now that we were upon our perpetrator, Shiela searched my van wildly with her frantic eyes. She found an old push broom handle behind the passenger seat, and leaped out of the van, beating the air with that stick she found. She screamed for the slick young Black man to stop, and at the same time, yelled for me to: "Get out and get him RahLeeCoh."

The young man, now an "alleged" thief, showed no fear as he crossed in front of my headlights. He moved with the confidence of someone knowledgeable of Criminal Law. With a sly grin on his face, and as cool as a cucumber, he chirped: "I was just playin' with y'all."

Well, despite Shiela's pleas, "I-was-not-about's-to-leave-my-position-behind-the¬wheel." I figured that all was well since we retrieved her car. Besides, I wasn't "packin" and my mechanical ram was ready to charge any aggressive move toward us. "I was not, as Martin would say-tryin' to be no police." The idea of risking my life further for some steel and plastic, did not appeal to me, especially since it can be replaced.

I mean anyway, hadn't I acted heroically enough already?! Had not I saved her precious little car?

Apparently, she did not feel that way. She wanted that "little so and so" put away. Evidently she did not agree with my logic, and I don't know if she ever forgave me for not making sure that the young fellow got punished for his crime. I do know that she did not thank me for saving her car, and neither she nor her husband ever came by to see the baby again (We did restore relations years later when our children attended middle school together).

Anyway, sorry about that little intrusion on our discussion about birth room preparations, but it was related to the help we got from our friends to ensure we were ready for the challenge of home childbirth.

Our friends helped us to feel that this was a special birthing. They realized, as we did, that, for the first time, we were taking our destiny in hand.

We felt like we were really ready, and we were encouraged for reasons other than the good feeling we got from our friends. The experience we gained from managing the birth of our previous son—Jolanti, provided us with the confidence that comes from first hand knowledge. So, we were not haunted by the feeling of uncertainty, nor plagued by occasional bouts with "old man fear."

The thing that was even more delightful for me was the fact that my wife finally came over to my position regarding her use of the services provided by local Women's Health clinics, medical doctors, and mid-wives. She no longer believed that they followed the soundest medical wisdom, or used correct and safe procedures. Thanks to my preaching and selection of literature on alternative medical approaches, she was persuaded by the medical reasoning, which justifies the health care and wellness theories advocated by Dr. Robert S. Mendelsohn, and other scholars such as Dr. Arnold Ehret, Dick Gregory, and Jethro Kloss. These theories-based on Health Teachings of Ancient Wisdom—contradict the theoretical foundation of practices used in contemporary prenatal and postnatal care.

This body of knowledge formed the basis of my objections to my wife's use of contemporary practitioners, but there were other reasons as well. The most objectionable was the manner in which these doctors in the medical facilities examined my wife. Their examination included the habit and practice of jabbing a finger up my wife's private place. (I didn't care if they were male or female; I was not in agreement wih this procedure.) In case you may be thinking that these doctors went to medical school to learn their craft, and I must be jealous. Well, I do love my wife very much, however, I base my objections on concrete evidence that exposes the inappropriateness of this procedure. It was painfully clear that each time the doctors used this procedure on my wife, they caused her to bleed, and left her in "hobbling" pain-pain that I had to relieve. (Our closeness, and my sensitivity caused her pain to be my pain; so I felt it too!)

Some may conclude that I don't possess the credentials to question modern medical practices, nor the training to judge the actions of modern medical doctors. But who can doubt the power of God, or the things that are possible through faith? My faith and trust in God led me to believe that the "finger jab" test was an unjustifiable and unholy intrusion into sacred territory. This belief evolved to the point where I viewed this tacky practice as the introduction of a potentially harmful element into the birthing equation. I came by these conclusions honestly. This viewpoint started to develop after the revelation I received in the back seat of a cab, when I witnessed the birth of our oldest daughter still living at home; Tashi, as we affectionately call her, crawled out of that birth canal, moving her hands and feet so fast that I thought I imagined something gray flying out under my wife's up-stretched legs. After I searched around and found her in the crevice of the back seat, I was struck with the immediate realization that God oversees natural births. Armed with this reality and proof of faith, I am filled with patience to wait until God reveals the miracle of new life. So, there is no reason for me to stick my finger into my wife's vagina, particularly since such an act increases the possibility that an unwanted foreign agent could slip into the canal on the finger (gloved or not). This agent could have ill intent for mother and child. The potential danger posed by such an unwarranted intrusion into the birthing canal takes precedence over any reasons we were offered to justify the use of said "fickle finger" test.

Since we are content to wait on God's confirmation and scheduled course of events, there is no need for me to use my fingers as a probing or measuring device to determine how many centimeters my wife has dilated. I know that I will be with her every minute; she is my only patient and there is no need to "hurry things along." So I don't have to break her waterbag (" . . . a common and safe procedure," says a doctor friend of our family. "Not so," I say. It may be common, but the "jury is in" concerning the issue of safety, especially in view of the high incidence of "code blue" condition created by this practice.) (Later, we look at the birthing story of our daughter-Rahkua, which took place in the so-called "Natural Birthing Wing" of a local Hospital. Not only does this story show how we arrive at our position condemning this practice, but it also reveals the reasons my wife became forever opposed to hospital births. In doing so, we also present the theory we developed about the negative effects and undesirable consequences resulting from the use of this procedure, including the "Code Blue" emergency procedures that can and do follow this bag breaking finger poking interference.)

None of the reasons our doctor friend gave us to justify such a procedure convinced me that such a "blood letting," pain causing, bag breaking, "code blue" condition creating, finger probing technique should be used on my wife, or any other expectant mother, for that matter. In fact, the previously mentioned experience gave me more reason to believe that it is very important for the bag to burst on its own. Our birthing experiences (a sampling of so little birthing data, without a control group, etc., may not be considered scientifically significant enough to warrant dependable conclusions, but we believe they are) lead us to believe that our theory is correct, and that, when the bag is ripe enough to burst, it does so, without outside help. This bursting power causes forces to mount further, and waters to rush. These cooperating movements work together to signal mom and babe to make the necessary efforts to separate from one another. We believe this happens naturally, when the time is right. We also believe that this is God's plan for the procreative process. For that reason, I am willing to wait for the baby to pop up and out of that glorious "P-hole;" to wait on God's unchanging hand!

I can wait to see whether my baby is a boy or girl. Then, I can go shopping for clothes, decide upon a name, or do any of the things that require knowledge of the precise gender of the baby.

I don't think that it is too wise to allow clothes and names and other such frivolous things that are not medical emergencies to dictate procedure and policy, or to "hurry along" a natural process.

The important point we make here is that we object to medical procedures that have basis in frail human values, and usurpation of power for non-medical reasons (see Male Practice). This includes methodology that is influenced by "vested interests," such as pharmaceutical companies, or insurance agencies that provide monetary incentives and other perks to promote their products and services. We will discuss the results of such non-medical intrusion upon the delivery process later, particularly a procedure instituted due to the powerful influence of King Louis XIV. For now, however, let us return to the discussion of the conditions surrounding the home birthing of our son, Rah-Imhotep,

Everything seemed to be going our way. Confident, and full of faith, we were certain about our plan, and we were familiar with all the steps to achieve our goal. All elements were ready, and in place, well in advance of the due date. We were clear about our actions, and "gung-ho" about getting all the pieces together just right. And, so we did.

Before we continue into our real life tale, lets briefly examine the steps we follow to get ready for our homebirth. For that purpose, we arrange all the elements involved in our preparation in a list that follows. Some of the items on this list may seem trivial. However, when you are "running around like a chicken with its head cut off," you will appreciate any relief to your tired back due to the fact that you paid close attention to the fine details. Even the smallest jobs executed at the point of delivery weigh heavily on your head, neck, back and mind. You will be glad that you considered every item.

ISHAKARAH FAMILY
HOME BIRTH PREPARATION LIST

- All clothes were washed, folded and stored
- All herb teas to be used were purchased, dry blended, labeled, and stored in a convenient location
- All floors were swept, scrubbed with soap and hot water, and disinfected
- The birthing room was cleaned, disinfected and organized
- A bundle of clean rags were placed under the bed
- A bundle of sheets were obtained, washed, wrapped in brown paper, and tied up (they were stored in readiness for baking in the oven prior to the last stages of delivery, for the purpose of sterilizing them)
- A clean mop and bucket were placed in a handy location
- The refrigerator was stocked, and, several meals were prepared and stored there, just before the due date-including plenty of fresh fruit, nuts, juices and bottled water enough to last a week
- The mattress was covered with plastic
- Changes of clothes for everyone to last 3 days were laid out, ironed and hung in easily accessible locations
- I arranged my free lance art business to accommodate a few days of "down time"
- We informed and received advice from some of our friends who happen to be physicians (including a Traditional Healer, under whom we studied certain aspects of the Healing Arts)
- We obtained appropriate literature to supplement our own collection—which we read and reread to one another on a regular basis
- We took early morning walks and late night strolls, sometimes with the entire family (these trips provided us with opportunity to collect aluminum cans, that gave birth to an exciting art form—aluminum spaceships and future automobiles, which are still awaiting acclaim)
- We obtained an ample supply of cloth diapers, and a complete collection of baby clothes and accessories for both sexes (Mamaku got more things for boys because she predicted (and correctly) that the baby was a boy; she based this on an "old time barometer," whereby the manner in which the baby protrudes in the belly, as well as the level of activity or movement the baby makes indicates the sex: boys are sluggish, and girls are active; boys lay high and pointed, girls develop low and rounded); the accessories included baby wipes, a nasal suction bulb, a breast pump, baby bottles, cotton swabs, safety pins, and Vaseline petroleum jelly

- We bought meditation and chant music cassette tapes
- We also purchased incense, candles, batteries, lamp oil, toiletries, and colored light bulbs

---

Once the above props were in place, the "stage was set" for our Rah-Imhotep birthing drama, which we begin from the point where I took my family to Greenville, MS.

Though Mamaku was very pregnant, we decided that this would be the last opportunity for her to get away. The Nelson Street Festival provided an opportunity for a business venture/vacation, where I could sell my T-shirt design, and other art, and give the family a welcomed change of scenery. This was also an excellent opportunity for me to introduce to Mississippi, the style of art I developed at the New Orleans Jazz and Heritage Festival a few years earlier, "Exact likeness Air Brush Portraits on T-shirts"—done on the spot.

Unfortunately for this business opportunity, the July heat was so unbearable that the small trickling crowd was not enough incentive to entice us to stay, and wait on sales. All we needed, to make up our mind, was a little mix-up about our booth location, and the threat of altercation with a tactless, inebriated vendor. This was our cue to leave that run down street that reflected unmerciful, baking rays from the sun. As I packed T-shirts, and custom brass ear-rings, and other crafts and fine art, I could not help but feel relief at the prospect of escaping what had begun to feel like a lost time capsule; it was as if Nelson Street 1992, had transformed into Hastings Street of Detroit in the 1950's, where the same drunken stupor hung in the air to numb the senses with visions of broken dreams, unrealized potentials, and smells from used bottles in brown paper bags, dangling from back pockets of area residents, who stumbled from last night's hangover into a never ending cycle of shady damp despair, that not even that blaring sun could dry out.

It was without regret that we retreated to the shade of the Hampton Inn, where we had spent the previous night, as the guests of one of the promoters of the festival. We had enjoyed our stay, and we were happy to return. We got some relief from the sun's blaring rays, in the big integrated swimming pool (a welcomed blessing in Mississippi), along with the barely used Jacuzzi, both of which refreshed and revived us. This was an ideal form of escape from the record breaking, 1992, 4th of July heat wave.

On our way back home to Jackson, we stopped in Belzoni, Mississippi, to see my Aunt Mary. It was a nice little visit, except for the giant mosquitoes that "gang raped" us, even in the daylight. We enjoyed our mini-vacation, eating Bar B Q fish, and freshly picked garden vegetables, and talking about the good old days, as we lounged in the cold atmosphere of air-conditioners turned up full blast. Even though we were having fun, we had to cut our visit short.

On the road, we were happy about our little unexpected vacation. We were also happy about something else. We got the chance to purchase our favorite summer food from a roadside fruit and vegetable stand-watermelon (we live up to stereotyping about southerners and watermelon; we love it with a passion and use it in healing therapies). The two delicious watermelons would remind us for several days, of our anxious journey through that long, lonely, flat, parched, and dusty Delta terrain.

Once we settled under the sanctuary of our own roof, I examined my wife. We were relieved to discover that the discomfort my wife experienced was not due to labor contractions. It appeared to stem from the fact that Baby-Cake (as he would come to be known) had shifted his position inside his mother's womb. His big head caused pressure pain and hindered Mamaku's circulation.

After completing the examination, I gave her an all over the body massage with olive oil. I rubbed into her bottom area, saturating and smoothing it in gently. My fingers carefully caressed her swollen belly, while I whispered sweet "some-things" into her and my unborn baby's ears.

I introduced some reflexology techniques at this point. I "worked on her feet," paying special attention to areas on the bottom of her feet that are physically and electro magnetically connected to the stressed and "labored" organs responsible for pregnancy and delivery. These foot massages brought the desired relief and much needed relaxation.

Over the next several days, our relaxed and satisfied state of mind allowed us to get totally prepared. Mamaku's enormous appetite, frequent trips to the "johnette," and focused "nesting" energy led us to judgment day. (Judgment day is an interesting choice of words, especially since it lets us add the fact that a most pressing factor influencing mama-to-be's state of mind during all these happenings was the trial proceedings that "hung" over our heads. The court adjourned her case, in which she defended herself against the double jeopardy retrying of facts already decided upon by the Mississippi Supreme Court (and the U.S. Supreme court in its silence), in her case (under her previous marriage name), McGlothin Vs The JPSD, whereby the original charge of "unprofessional attire"-meaning head wraps and headcoverings, as "written" grounds for dismissal, were altered to a "verbal" charge of "dirty, filthy, Dredlock hair, with particles of lint in it"-which was a painful untruth, and new grounds for the same old unlawful dismissal Judge Fred Banks ruled as violation of McGlothin's First Amendment Rights; it was adjourned until after the delivery. We were handling the unjustness of the situation as bravely as possible, but this, without a doubt was additional burden on her pregnant mind. Coincidently enough, Akua's attorney at the time (she had a few others throughout the eight year ordeal), "threw" a party, on the day before the date of the delivery.

We took the whole family to the political party, happy to share in a festive atmosphere, which we felt would be our last chance to be out together for "a good little while." We were right! This was count down, as the unfolding adventure reveals!

When we returned home from the party, the children fell asleep, "as soon as their heads hit the pillow." Their bellies were full, and they were exhausted from dancing, playing, and partying with their parents and a broad cross section of Jackson's citizenry, including people of different races, young people, old people, other children, another pregnant mother, politicians, attorneys, business and common folks. They had a full day and evening of fun and excitement.

The next day was just as full and emotionally draining. So, after a morning full of friends coming by to visit, as if spiritually sent to bless our birthing and welcome the coming of new life and a new family member, I put the children to bed (an interesting factual tidbit: an African gentleman informed me that a term for delivery in the Mother-land is "put to bed"); this was done around 1:OOPM.

Mamaku went into the bathroom. She had the urge to clear out her bowels, and take a warm bath.

Meanwhile, I went into the bedroom, lit some incense, and turned on a soft blue light. I also put on a cassette tape, and played soothing *chant* music.

Then, I went into the kitchen, to brew a special blend of herb tea. It was a pregnancy blend that Mamaku created; it contained Red Raspberry, Squaw-vine, and Valerian Root. (You may consult Dr. Kloss, in "Back To Eden," for information regarding the properties of these and other herbs, including the correct way to prepare, and use herb tea.) I brought an iron pot of water to a boil, before extinguishing the fire. I added a tablespoon of Mamaku's pregnancy blend to the boiling water immediately after I cut off the fire, covered the pot with a saucer, and allowed the tea to steep for a few minutes.

By this time, a peaceful and healing air filled the house. The sweet smells of herbs and fragranted oils floated in the air, which was lit up with blue hues and colorful echoes. I wanted the atmosphere to be just right for Mamaku, who was just coming out of the bathroom.

I decided to take a bath myself, so I went into the bathroom and began removing my clothes. Before I could climb into the tub, I was startled by Mamaku's screaming words: "Baba, I think the baby is gonna come now, . . . you better get me up quick!"

I turned, stark naked, and ran back into our bedroom, which we converted into a birthing room. I raced to the bed, which Mamaku had rearranged with the rest of the furniture, as she single handedly ordered the room, flipping the mattress and also, disinfecting everything.

I quickly reached the foot of the bed, where Mamaku sat in her favorite Zen position. I got behind her, slipped my hands under her armpits, and lifted her onto the bed.

All of a sudden, without warning, a burst of water (amniotic fluid) drenched me, and the bottom portion of our mattress; it was exposed, as I struggled to hoist Mamaku up onto the bed. Our carefully laid plans began to fade, when our abrupt actions disturbed the old sheets and plastic covering we hoped would provide protection. Water "slushed," and "gushed" all over our shiny hardwood floor, the thoughtful little area rug, and my naked body.

This unexpected dash on our detailed preparations caused me to become a bit unsettled. Yet, I managed to pull and haul Mamaku further up, into the bed. In doing so, I began to worry. I wondered if the lugging, and tugging and contorted position of Mamaku's body would have a negative effect upon the baby's ability to push up and out of his mother. My thoughts became frantic, as I imagined that his job could be hindered by the absence of lubricating fluid, and lack of the "flushing" action, which just occurred.

Mamaku was surprisingly calm, despite my mounting inner turmoil. She did not seem to share my unmentioned concern. In fact, she was surrounded by a strange, and peaceful glow. "This was a good thing," too, because she had to point to the places we stored everything. My mind suddenly refused to know anything! It was also a good thing that Mamaku had regained her composure so quickly and remarkably. This minor miracle immediately infected me. I recaptured control over my senses.

I was strengthened by Mamaku's trust in me, and I began praying silently. I used my hands to relieve my wife's pain, as I assisted both of the bodies depending on me to perform their respective tasks. This meant giving a deep penetrating, yet gentle massage.

I began speaking soft, soothing words to both mother and unborn child, and the contractions got closer and closer. Stronger, and stronger grew the eruptions of "Mount Vagina." Louder and louder grew the moans and groans. Until, finally, a wrinkled gray mass appeared. It filled the open human crevice-showing through like the tip top of an old bald headed man's crown. Things had begun to move, as if in rapid slow motion, and just as quickly as the mass appeared, it bubbled up equally as fast.

It was the baby's head! It "slooshed" out, and fell over limply. A horrific sight shook my senses; the umbilical cord was wrapped around my baby's neck!

Fear gripped me. It applied even more pressure on my emotional sensibilities, which were already tested, jarred and frantic.

With a chipper outward guise, I hid the frightening sight from my wife. I did not think that I should let her know that I couldn't tell whether or not the baby was alive! I couldn't possibly tell her that the tiny little big head lay bent over, limp and blue gray in color. As calmly as I could, I reached under the cord, and flipped it over the baby's head. The head came up; pushed out by the undeniable force of the emerging shoulders. Then, because the torso came up next, I could see that "self," that "peeda," and the sight caused me to yell: "It's a boy! . . . I have another son!"

It was not until then that he began to gasp, gurgle, and cry. Only then were my tortured emotions relieved. I thanked God and Mamaku, expressing my joy out loud.

I felt good, as I clamped the cord, placing one clamp an inch and a half from the baby's belly, and the other clamp, an inch from that point. (These measurements were, of course, approximations determined by "eyeing.") Then, I cut the cord with the sterilized blade, also provided by our friend Shiela. This was all done as Rah—Imhotep rested on his mother's thigh, while her hands covered and warmed his big fat body.

He was the biggest of our babies. Weighing over ten pounds, he had a butt that started at his shoulders and ended at his ankles.

At that moment, the doorbell rang. I placed 'Hotep in his mother's arm, and planted a wet kiss on her waiting lips. Then, I hurried to the front door, with visions of the indescribable loving look in Mamaku's eyes competing for attention in my mind, with the memory of the sensual feeling her grateful hands left in a soothing trail from my arm, down to my tired finger tips. When I reached the door, I peeped through the curtains to see Nikki Jean.

I was still naked, so I spoke to Nikki Jean through the door. I instructed her to come in, lock the door behind herself, and come back to the bedroom. Then, after I unlocked the door, I took off, running down the hallway, before she could enter our front room.

By the time Nikkie Jean reached the bedroom, I had put on some clothes. She strolled curiously into our personalized birthing wing. She smiled at the wonderful sight that greeted her when her eyes focused on the miracle laid out before her in that warm blue atmosphere. She was just in time to witness me cleaning and dressing the fat little fellow. I was satisfied that 'Hotep passed inspection, and I passed him over to Nikki Jean, after she had washed up. She was delighted, and the two of them bonded for a short while, before she handed him to his mother-who "nursed" him to sleep.

When I finished mopping the floor, and cleaning up myself and the surrounding areas, I made some Penny Royal herb tea, and brought a cup to

Mamaku. Then, we began to wait for the placenta to deliver. We got a little uneasy, because of the memory of the late delivery experience we had in our last birthing of our son Jolanti. Our worries were unfounded, because in less than twenty minutes that phase of the birthing came to pass too.

Since we believe in the biblical passage extolling the cleansing virtue of Hyssop, we not only drank said herb tea, but we also included some into the wet rag bath of Baby-Cake.

Mamaku-adhering to her hometown (Meridian, MS) upbringing, wherein the new mother receives instructions not to get wet all over-also took a localized "squat" bath. She did so using liquid peppermint soap and the hyssop tea. She was forced to do this because Baby-Cake demonstrated his gratitude by showering his mother with a thick, sticky, tar colored "booboo" that refused to rub off without much work (Hey that reminds me of the movie Jason's Lyric, where the "wine-head-looking-alley-preacher" squalled out his prophetic observation: "They got shit in the world . . . you can't rub it off." Anyone who is "up on" the chronology of these events-the movie and this birthing-must realize that this last little intrusion is only possible because I enter it as I execute my sixth draft of this manuscript on October 11, 2000. Throughout this written adventure we include such literary jumps in and out of time periods, hopefully to the reader's delight. Now, let us return to the past.)

It is late night, just after mid-night, Friday, June 7, 1996, and I am forced to interrupt our story of Rah-Imhotep's birthing. In fact, I'll quickly bring it to a close, in order that we may discuss the reason that I am so very excited at this time of night.

In conclusion, I must say that I was very relieved and pleased that mother and child were safe and healthy. Baby-Cake looked straight into my eyes, he had all his fingers and toes, he could hear, and he was not clogged with mucus. Mamaku too, seemed strong and sound thanks to the herb teas, regular walks, massages, and exercise. She did not tear, but she did complain of a burning sensation in her "taint." And, lastly, the placenta came out cleanly, and intact. All was well, as I took a quiet moment to sit and gaze at the holy sight of my wife and our newborn son.

I watched, as the old and new loves of my life fell asleep. We were alone, now, and they were exhausted. They made such a heavenly picture, clinging to one another, sharing the warm soothing feelings generated by suckling lips, and gentle fingers that trigger womb tightening contractions. "Yeah, yeah," I know you are saying . . . "that's nice, but what about that exciting news?"

Well, O.K., let's just call it an "instant story," and, it is presently unfolding, even as I write. The story concerns my wife's latest revelation-reception of a sensitive climax, and fitting end to our most recent joint book reading adventure: "I Tituba, Black Witch Of Salem." (Tituba's fateful end left us in pain, and in need of a more just finale to the story.)

We will use this timely "instant story" as a jumping off point, which will allow us to ease right on into our next chapter, which deals with our observations of events and circumstances unique to the instant, evolving birth, and promising gift of life for our family.

And so the story goes . . . . :

I was outside, on our front porch, enjoying the cool Mississippi night air, as I played the strings of the "harp looking" structure I retrieved from an old discarded piano. I was creating music using Popsicle sticks, soothing myself in a rare moment of solitude. I had put the children to bed. The peaceful mood of the house inspired me to release my spirit using my improvised musical instrument, which produced a kind of symphonic harp/kettle drum type of meditative sound. I created musical vibrations that flowed rhythmically on the wings of Mississippi fireflies, and moonbeams that bathed my wife and me in an ancient mystical light. It was just the right background for the poetic words that my wife began to share with me.

At first, I thought the words were those of Maryse Conde-the author of the book, which my wife and I started reading several weeks back. However, there was something about the words she was reading that mirrored my feelings, and the spiritual connection between the three of us-my wife, Tituba, and myself. It was the kind of "something" that the author couldn't possibly have known. It was a personal and private empathy that exploded into realization. As my hands strummed the old piano strings, the vibrations accompanied words that I now realized were my wife's own heart murmurs. We created a night concert of powerful, healing words and musical notes-an acclamation of my wife's graduation into the ranks of great Mississippi writers, like William Faulkner, and Alice Walker.

Akua's (Mamaku's) timely and spiritually inspired words provided us both with a just ending to a tragic story of persecution-a persecution we both endure and feel because of our love for people, our embrace of the healing arts (which is what we believe the so-called witches really practiced), and our passion for fair play and justice.

When Mamaku came out, I didn't hear all her words at first, because I was so preoccupied with creating rhythmic musical patterns, in hopes of catching a melody. I knew she was reading about Tituba. I just figured she was reading an Epilogue by Maryse. After a while the words sunk in and rose from my subconscious perception to conscious understanding. I then realized that the excellent prose I was hearing had to be my wife's own literary offerings. I requested her to reread those beautiful words, because bass and treble clef vibrations had drowned out some of them.

45

Before she began over, I took pause, and received her permission to name her journalistic inspiration: "Song For Tituba." (See Appendix B, for a copy.)

When Akua started rereading "her story," our interdisciplinary concert of music and literature was on! We went to a "grooving" zone, and had a glorious and self-fulfilling climax. We synchronized in spiritual release, and came together in a harmony of grammatical soul sounds, and pure musical vibes, drifting and floating on a cool late night Mississippi breeze.

The instant we reached our inspired improvisational finale, I called Mamaku my Queen. I professed to her that her sensitive depth of literary and journalistic talent would soon be recognized and rewarded. Then, I proceeded to fall to my knees, bowing to her, as she grinned and blushed.

Hey, . . . that's cute, but, what in the heaven were we talking about?

Oh yeah, . . . we were about to conclude our discussion on Birth Room Preparations and Readiness, when we got side tracked by the sound of our own horn tooting.

Please focus your attention back on the points we covered in this chapter, which reveal the way we got ready, and prepared for our last son's birth.

We concentrated on things we did to prepare our bedroom, such as clean, order, sanitize, and stock (in an easily accessible place) all tools, and supplies for delivery. We also talked about the things that made us ready. This included keeping Mamaku in a positive, and peaceful mental state, with an oiled, massaged and exercised body, as well as, maintaining a strict dietary regimen. We mentioned that her diet contained an abundance of fresh fruit, and vegetables, and specific herb tea consumption. However, we failed to note the importance of vitamin/mineral supplementation.

We won't get into a long and drawn out story about it. But, early in that pregnancy, it was clear that "ole" 'Hotep was eating up all of his mother's bodily supply of vitamin and minerals. She became weak, and exhausted. She also suffered from excruciating toothaches. This condition disappeared immediately, once we introduced a pregnancy vitamin/mineral supplement to her daily intake.

We also tried to get across the idea that, even though your "well laid" plans may cover everything, you would do well to expect the unexpected, and maintain a level head, fortified by trust in God.

Before we could finish our thought, we found ourselves in the grips of an instant story that had to be told. This notion of capturing an event as it occurs, aptly sets the stage for the next chapter, which exploits the idea of keeping an instant record of the birthing preparations that we follow in this immediate pregnancy, as we describe and explain its evolvement.

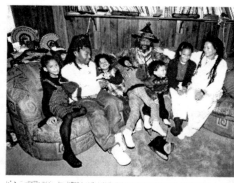

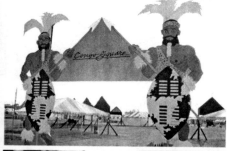

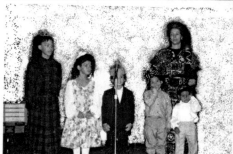

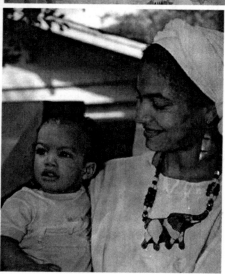

Top left: Rahkua; Aahtahbah; Rah-Imhotep; RahLeeCoh Jolanti; Baba RahLeeCoh; Namibiyah; Tashi; and Mama Akua pregnant with Rahzizi in 1995 by Ptah

Top right: The 1988 Entrance Façade RahLeeCoh created for the Congo Square section of the New Orleans Jazz and Heritage Festival (two twenty foot Zulu Warriors)

Bottom left: Tashi, Rahkua, Jolanti, Rah-Imhotep, grandson Jaylon with Mama Akua leading off the Kwanzaa celebrations photo by Daisy Garrett (digitally enhanced by RahLeeCoh)

Bottom right: RahLeeCoh Jolanti being held by his mother in 1992

47

CHAPTER 4

DAILY RECORD OF PRESENT PREGNANCY

In this chapter, we hope to be more scientific; particularly regarding data collection, even though we feel the act of childbirth is essentially a spiritual phenomenon. We begin by presenting the story that led to this fresh approach to record keeping, that ultimately shows how we manage our lives (our life style) during Mamaku's pregnancy. By approaching data collection through the use of a daily log of events, circumstances, and important facts, we establish a record of the steps we generally follow to reach our goal of a successful home birth. This daily log, for the most part is made up of a series of short stories. These stories, written while they are fresh, illustrate how, and why we take certain steps, as we describe and analyze said procedures. We view the results and consequences of our actions through glimpses of mental and physical changes, as well as verbal pictures of reactions to events occurring during the period of pregnancy, as these events and actions unfold. We also devise a chart to record mental, and physical changes, note pregnancy problems, complaints and solutions, and list food selection and menus.

But, first let's get to our story that led to the idea of immediate data collection. And, like Greer used to say on "In Living Color:" "If you want to hear it, here it go!"

It is Tuesday night, 11:35PM, and we are feeling good about our family hour with friends. We are all on the front porch, enjoying this cool Mississippi night air again. We are communing with one another's souls, touching each other's feelings, and boosting self-esteem, as we share love in the night.

After our friends left, as we made our way back into the house, I touched and squeezed Mamaku's big belly. I noted the roll of flab circling her swollen womb, and I mentioned it to her. I was immediately filled with the urge to go write more in this little birthing book.

I became consumed by a great brainstorm. I got the urgent idea to begin recording pertinent facts surrounding this unfolding pregnancy.

(We interrupt this story with a "now" family happening. The children just called me into their room to show me their tent. They constructed it by draping two sheets over the foot of two beds, with a chair holding up the center. They were proud and happy about their accomplishment, smiling, and crawling in and out of the cozy little cubby. I smiled, and complimented them on their ingenuity. I marveled at their unpretentious and innocent fun. After absorbing this happy moment for a "short while," I walked back up front to secure the house for the night. As I did, I thought about Aahtahbah-my first born. She had constructed a similar tent for us to snuggle under, nearly ten years ago, in Thibodaux, Louisiana, at her Grandmother's house. The feeling of missing her overwhelmed me, so I paused for a pensive and relaxing moment, with a seat on the front porch swing. I began to contemplate the events surrounding the birth of "all my children"-no pun on the "soap" intended. Finally I thought about the fact that I am an Artist, yet I have not drawn sketches of any of my babies while they are developing in their mother's womb.

I was immediately filled with the urge to begin a graphically illustrated record of the various stages of Mamaku's physical changes. So I thought: "When I get back to the bedroom, I will draw a charcoal pencil sketch of Mamaku's nude body, to record this stage of her pregnancy."

However, by the time I secured the house for the night, and made it back to the bedroom, the urge to draw was replaced by the desire to write, which I had begun doing before the children called me into their room.)

Excuse me for that intrusion, but, if you know children, you know that they will repeat what they want of you, over and over and over again, until you give in, or go fly over the Cuckoo's nest with Jack Nicholson.

Anyway, let's back up a little, so we can talk about what has occurred thus far in this pregnancy. We'll start from the beginning, catch up to the present, and then begin to keep a current and running record.

It all began when Mamaku and the five of our children who live at home with us, returned from Meridian. This trip was compliments of her sister, who gave Mamaku and our five babies a little vacation back to their hometown, for a few days. I remained home with a grin on my face. I was very happy at the prospect of getting some peace and solitude. I was elated by the idea of being alone for the first time since I took on the responsibility of making and raising a family.

As you might have guessed, I was just as happy when they returned home to me. This occurred four days after they left. When my sister-in-God's-law, brought my family back, there was a different look in her eyes—a more appreciative, more understanding look. She was obviously happy to be relieved of her duty. Mamaku was obviously happy for me to take control of the reigns, and I was happy the solitude and blaring silence was over, and my family was back, safe and sound.

You might say that Mamaku and me were too happy to be back together, because we got carried away. She let her guard down. I didn't wear a "prophylactic jacket," and she didn't use the rhythm method. So, . . . showered by my satiated and grateful rain of human being seeds, a "child flower," fertilized with our love, is now growing in her "womb garden."

I am pretty certain that she is pregnant, because we have seen all of the signs that convince me of impregnation—as discussed in Chapter 2, which serve as my "Babyometer."

Yet, whenever I speak about our coming "infant crop," Mamaku denies that she is pregnant. Perhaps she is doing this in reaction to comments made by some of our "well meaning" friends, who seem to feel close enough to let her know that they disapprove of her having anymore babies. Some of these so called friends—and I hope they really are—have Expressed the opinion that they feel my wife and me are too old to be having children. (She is forty-three, and I will be fifty on the fourth of July, this year, 1996.)

I say: "What about Sarah, . . . and, doesn't God know bestl?"

Regardless of what "they" say, our faith in God is strong, and, we are committed to the healing principles that ensure protection for our obedience to divine will when it comes to being fruitful and multiplying. A few issues related to questions centering on our age do go through my mind, though. Yet, I feel that I am in good shape, especially since the girls in my High School-Ecorse High, in Ecorse, Michigan, made sure that I remained a virgin, until I left for college. Thanks to those girls, I did not waste my sperm. More importantly, my wife did not abuse her sex organs either (so she says, . . . and, . . . I believe her too, really, ... I do.)

So, here we are, old, yet young, because, neither did we destroy our body temple with alcohol and drugs (I can still remember the time I was introduced to marijuana. We were at a party, and a couple of friends discretely pulled out a "joint." When I came out with a loud: "Oough, yall smoking that stuff," my friends who were 4.0 college students, at WSU, and who *had* thought I was "cool," flew away from me, like I was a "square" who had contracted the Bubonic Plague), nor did we "over consume" nutritionally devitalized foods. Instead, we chose to make green leaf vegetables and the herbs of the field our meat, as advised in Genesis 1:29 & 30. Further, our youth-though we grew up in different areas of the nation, during different eras of time-was not filled with promiscuity (in my case it wasn't because I didn't want "it," it had more to do with the fact that I was fat and smart, and my Daddy had tight reigns on me). We did not "caste our sperm (or eggs) upon the waterbeds" of too many fruitless affairs.

Our reward comes now, late in life, when we are fruitful; God blesses us with beautiful children (I am not "tripping," but they look like pretty little doll children.). It seems that our abstinence in youth allowed us to multiply in our later years. It also seems that now, all we have to do is touch each other with a kiss, and Mamaku gets pregnant! (She has been known to tell people that she is really a virgin, and every time we try to "do it," she gets pregnant; or, she tells them that she has only "done it" the amount of times that we have children.)

Meanwhile, as I stated, since that "womb-planting-happy-home coming," I have observed all the signs of pregnancy.

Several interesting things have occurred in our lives, since that point of conception. They affect Mamaku's state of mind, and disposition; I believe they have an influence on our baby's development and growth. First, Mamaku left her position as teacher, for a local A.M.E. Church Day Care Center. Secondly, we both were selected as "extras" in the movie, "Ghost Of Mississippi," staring Whoppi Goldberg (It was filmed downtown). Together these two events mark a significant point in this pregnancy, and that has to do with money. Now that we have spent all the money from our little acting debut, and Mamaku received her final check from her teaching services, I must become more creative in the ways I earn money. (I was more equipped to do this before I "came-down-with" the symptoms Sinbad jokes about, when he describes the "Brother" who gets married, and has his brains sucked out, leaving him with a blank look, wandering aimlessly around Malls, carrying packages.)

I would prefer this money to come from my art creativity, productions and commissions. However, now, such opportunities seem to avoid my sluggish attempts to generate new business, or hold onto old business relations of the past. My old "hustles" (like, on the spot portrait drawing, custom signs and brass ear ring sales, lecture/demonstrations, exhibitions, grants, etc.), seem to have become dinosaur baggage. This has placed a burden on our ability to purchase the expensive dietary, and nutritional supplements, and other such Health Food Store needs.

God is great, though, and as we speak, a corner lot full of big healthy Dandelion greens have been provided for us. Most folks consider these herbs of the field as weeds (Please consult "BackTo Eden," to discover the unbelievable number of health benefits you get from eating this free growing herb.)

After we harvested a great deal of this Dandelion crop, I could hardly wait for my wife to turn those so called weeds into one of the best tasting meal ever eaten, by King or pauper.

Mamaku did not let us down; she created a Dandelion stew that was certain to be a storehouse of vitamins and minerals that promised to make Mama and our unborn, healthy and strong. The Dandelions were the main dish of that splendid dinner, which was garnished and flavored with other herbs and spices. It was so good that I had to share it with an old lady friend of our family, who lives behind us, on the next street. She too had the same enthusiastic reaction to that unique, fresh taste my wife achieved.

This meal is indicative of the kind of food choices that have characterized Mamaku's diet so far, in this pregnancy. That diet has also included fresh juice from sweet potatoes, turnip green roots and leaves, carrots, and apples. These were all juiced in our Champion juicer, which we obtained seventeen years ago, upon Dick Gregory's recommendation, in his book, "Cooking With Mother Nature-For Folks Who Eat." Since that time, fresh juice has become an integral part of our diet.

We will get into a more detailed look at our dietary plan later (including the food consumption choice for the entire family). But, first we have arranged a list of all the foods that comprise our basic intake thus far in this pregnancy.

Ishakarah Family Dietary Intake In The Instant Pregnancy

- Beans and Peas (We love all kinds of the both of these, but Mamaku usually eliminates these from our diet early in her pregnancy. Folk tale has it, that beans make the baby's bones hard, which could make delivery difficult.)

• Greens	* Carrots	* Water Melon (as much as possible)
• Apples	* Lemons	* Oat Meal & Corn Meal
• Bananas	* Sea Weeds	* Oven Baked Corn Bread (herbal)
• Grapes	* Soy Margarine	* Tomatoes
• Raisins	* Oranges (lots)	* Wheat Bread
• Pineapples	* Peppers	* Wheat Crackers
• Coconuts	* Ketchup	* Cayenne
• Brown Rice	* Brewers Yeast	* Olive Oil
• Grapefruit	* Cashew Butter	* Texturized Vegetable Protein
• Fish	* Tuna fish	* Corn
• Celery	* Honey	* Broccoli
• Nuts	* Pop Corn	* Bell Peppers
• Potatoes	* Onions	* Mushrooms

As you can see, except for the food we didn't include—cookies, ice cream, potato chips, candy and Dark Beers, the consumption of which we blame on the children-the foods on our preceding list indicate the fact that our meals are prepared from scratch, for the most part.

We may joke about our slips and departures from what we believe is the healthiest way to eat, but we know that good health is no laughing matter, and that there is nothing nutty about a person who is concerned about their health and well being. Therefore, our minds remain focused, even though we may get weak sometimes, and backslide. Nevertheless, we remain steadfast in our vow not to eat flesh (we haven't slipped that much), and our intention is to regain, and maintain a strict vegetarian way of life. (**"By and Large,"** we believe in Dr. Arnold Ehret's position, which is that optimum wellness comes from eating a diet of foods that do not produce mucus, such as green leaf vegetables, fruit, and nuts.)

In addition to the foods mentioned, our diet thus far in this present pregnancy has also included trips to The Restaurant Salad Bar. Though our finances have been "challenged," this pregnancy, we've managed to feed the family with salads from The Restaurant on a few occasions. For around $5.00, we could purchase two prepackaged garden salads, and one crab salad from the well-stocked salad bar-where Mamaku would "load up" and pack the containers to the bursting point. She and I would split the one from the salad bar, and we would divide the prepackaged ones between the children. I think that perhaps we put too much pressure on that salad bar, by feeding our family in such a manner. I don't know if any other families were doing the same thing, but I do know that The Restaurant changed their self serve policy when it came to that salad bar. They started handing only the bottom portion of the container to the salad bar customer. The top and bag were then only available after the bottom was filled and returned to the counter. So our creative feeding came to an end. It was just as well though, because-though the green salads at The Restaurant were great—that crabmeat certainly was not the "herb bearing plants of the field." It actually falls into the classification of mucus causing foods identified by Dr. Ehret. Thus, eating it means a departure from the meaning of strict vegetarianism. (It was this same commitment to not eating meat, plus the fact that we abhor injustice, that made my wife and me "long" to go to Texas, to add our support to Oprah's legal battle with the Beef Barons.)

Speaking of not being strict, and staying on a "mucusless" diet program, as I mentioned, when Mamaku interrupts our usually healthy diet with overwhelming cravings for junk food, and odd combinations of food, at crazy times of the day, I am convinced that she is pregnant. So far this pregnancy, she has sent me out for chocolate nut candy bars, and egg foo young, shrimp/pickle combinations. The other night, at 2:00 A.M., she craved Pop Corn, and Brewer's Yeast. Today, June 13, 1996, she acted like she could kill for peaches (even green ones), with salt sprinkled over them.

At this point, we have examined the factors that have a significant bearing on our procreative evolvement thus far, and we have caught up to the present. From this point forward, we shall maintain a detailed daily log of events, as they occur. To assist our efforts, we devised a chart to record relevant information, and keep track of changes in Mamaku's progress. We provide a sample of this chart, including a completed one, in the Appendix.

Now without further ado, we begin our narrative log of daily events significant to this instant pregnancy, on this, the 14th day of June 1996.

53

Today was great, unlike yesterday-when Mamaku complained of a neck ache and irritability. Today, she was active. She went walking, and took a shopping trip with our daughter, Nzinga. She was happy, and in a "loving" mood. She became very amorous, so much so, that I must share those delicious feelings (which may have been a dream?).

Mamaku slipped on some tights. They were black, with little straps that hooked under her feet. She covered these with a thin "wrap" skirt, which was bright, with abstract flower designs lit up all over. Loose fitting, and split up the center, the skirt swayed and mesmerized like a Hawaiian Moon Dance.

I was sitting on the porch swing, tired from a busy day of cleaning the house, washing dishes and a load of clothes, retrieving a sixteen foot ladder from a friend, walking to the Auto Zone Parts Store-to purchase a "pick-up-coil" to repair our Ford Escort, and taking care of some Art business. Worn down, I was relaxing away the stress of the day, lounging on the porch, nodding and drifting.

Presently, as if floating in a hazy dreamy vision, Mamaku sauntered smoothly over toward me. She had a mischievous grin plastered over her face. I soon discovered the source of her sneaky little secret. The grin on her face grew, like the fun she was having watching my reaction to her unfolding drama. It grew bigger and bigger, radiating with a playful and provocative glow.

When Mamaku got close to me, she quickly lifted her left leg, and did a slow motion "round house" karate kick . . . right over my unsuspecting head! I did not have time to marvel at her beautiful martial-arts form and focused control, because I was pleasantly surprised and startled by such a sight!

The colorful dress fell away from her up stretched leg, revealing black tights that had a slit, straight down the middle of the crotch! I was teased by a quick contrasting vision of "pink-eyed frilly black sweetness," sandwiched in creamy colored softness, framed by the velvety blackness of the tights. "Talkin' bout a black tight sight. Man!"

"My picture was taken" by wide-open lips, draped in swiggly black excitement. It was a picture of instant arousement. (Hey, that made me think of Shaka Zulu. He would "parade" naked women through his vast number of troops, and if that "thang" rose up, it got chopped off! Ouch!)

Anyway, once we reached the bedroom, I was being led, like a mule reaching for that illusive carrot. In this case, the "carrot" was an "all-seeing-self-reproductive-eye," that charmed and lured me until I couldn't stand it anymore.

However, after I lay in bed, my erected senses were rebuffed. So, all I could do was turn over, as I thought: "Well, I need to be strong anyway, because, didn't the "21st Century Survival Handbook" state that pregnant, or lactating mothers should not be aroused or enticed; . . . and, didn't Ra Un Nefer Amen proclaim that intercourse beyond six times a year robs the body of essential vitamin/mineral count, that cannot be replaced? (See "Health Teachings Of The Ancient Wisdom.") "Yeah," I thought, "but, Mamaku was the one who initiated this; . . . she was the one who had "led a horse to water and wouldn't let him drink."

I must have drifted off to sleep for a moment, because I was shaken into awareness by a pleasing surprise. I was being carried away on a wave of pleasure. It felt like a tide of ecstasy, bent on rhythmic release. It crested and fell, crested and fell, deliriously building poetic motions of "squeezed eyed love visions," that were so accommodating and so fulfilling. But, just as we were about to "wipe out" in an emotional flood of pure *climaxic* delight, the door to the bedroom began to squeak open, ever so slowly.

I was not sure if I were awakening from a dream, yet in a husky, air catching gulp, I admonished our youngest son. I reminded Rah-Imhotep that he should always knock, and be given permission, before entering a closed door.

Having such dreamy pleasure interrupted, it seemed to be an impossibility to recapture the magic. So, we gave in to the host of little heads that began peeping, and popping around the open door. Their little brother—the "point man," had blazed the trail and led the way. So, we decided to let them in, and watched a video movie, which we rented the night before, from the Fortification Street Jitney Jungle, where we get our fresh fruit, when we can't make it to the Farmer's Market, or want to venture past the Capitol Street Jitney.

You may be wondering how this little episode relates to a positive pregnancy for Mamaku. The calm state she appears to be in at this time has to have a healing effect on her total being. In addition, the beautiful words of appreciation that flow from my heart must surely ease her easily troubled mind. With those sweet utterances, I kissed and nibbled on her hurts and pains. There was an expression of almost unbearable fulfillment written on her face.

Those heartfelt words must have been meant for Mamaku only; I wanted to share them, but I can't recall them.

It is a day later, and I'm still unable to recall those special words that whispered through me, flowing into Mamaku's ears, eyes, and face. I want to recall those special words so much so that I'm considering going into meditation to bring them back. The wonderful reflection they made in Mamaku's appearance is reason I want to remember them. She appears to radiate like a vision of eternal calmness and blissful love.

It may sound funny, but those beautiful words actually felt healing to me, as they left my lips. I can remember expressing to my wife, in the after math of our bliss, that her compelling sensuality made me want to confess, like an alter boy, to a Catholic Priest. We laughed together, because she knew that I was "poking fun" at her religious background. She also knows that, like me-raised as a "Northern-influenced-down¬Home-Southern-Baptist-she too, now embraces an "All-Faith" Theology.

What a glorious day is Father's Day of 1996!

We were just awakened like a "ping," 'Hotep just burst into our bedroom with his usual "heart pulling" bid for attention. Mamaku left with him. They left me alone, sitting and writing about this glorious morn . . . And, like a "ping," I was awakened again. This time, it was a cup of cucumber juice. Mamaku followed this "one," with a "two" punch-a cup of freshly juiced carrot juice, only moments later.

The cold, sweet and delicious carrot juice got my creative roller coaster moving.

Then, the doorbell rang, with the promise of a coming productive adventure. It was our spiritual sister-Dahli. You remember her, the lady who was involved in the "Ninja-Mama-Episode" that we mentioned in the Preface. This sensitive sister brought the "Sunday Morning Service" to us. She even brought a "member" with her, as well as the message, and the question we would ponder, and jointly answer, as we received the inspired words.

The subject of our impromptu spiritual session concerned: "What is the prerequisite for a man's state of mind, that makes it possible for him to cultivate and harvest his own human seed?" And, "What principles, and beliefs can he rely upon to direct his mind and hands to bring forth his own child?"

Of course, I didn't know all the facts just stated, at the time the doorbell rang, and we received our guests. I (we) became aware gradually, as the following recollection reveals.

I dressed quickly, paying little attention to style. As I did, I noticed that one of my Dred Locks was standing straight up, at attention. It was obviously revived, and energized by the handful of cucumber juice I rubbed into my scalp, and massaged into my hair. When I reached the front porch, I was pleasantly surprised to find Brother Paule sitting on the swing. He too was ready, and in need of a "culturally-religious, and spiritual communion."

Mamaku returned from within the house carrying a "Boom-Box," and a cassette tape, which she played at once. The tape contained a musical sound that gave the impression of a "Universal-Carribean-Raegae-Soulful-Rap,"-a delightful, freehearted feeling of love.

I was astonished, and happy to discover that Paule produced that wonderful tape. I was honored to learn that he wanted me to add some bamboo flute "licks" to the tune, to give it more of an exotic flare. Mamaku explained this to me, as she handed me one of the many bamboo flutes that I make. And, . . . we were off and running.

I tuned into the spirit that caused melodies and "licks" (this is a musician's term for receiving, and playing a set of musical notes related in a specific rhythm pattern of time and harmonic progression; usually one "hears" one's own instrumental part, which fits and accompanies a particular "riff," or composition) to flow through me, and out of the carefully drilled, smoothed, burned and sanded holes in the bamboo sections. My accompaniment sound was right on time!

This further "juvenated" my spirits, as the thought crossed my mind of how blessed our Nation is to have a President who is able to tune into and receive improvisational saxophone licks. He does this on a professional level, in one of the most sophisticated forms of music on the Planet-Jazz.

Then, I got the urge to play my trombone (I am not as accomplished as our President, but I do alright.), so, I jumped up, and ran toward the back room, where I kept my horn stored. While running down the hall to retrieve my ax (a musician's term given to a musical instrument) melodic "licks" filled my mind's ear.

As I hurried back up the hall to the porch, playing my little "ditty" over and over, until I had it *down pat*. Confident that I could play it correctly, I burst out of the front door. The door swung open wide, and I leaped into the air. When I landed on my two feet, I leveled my trombone, aiming it toward the passing cars. Suddenly, bold, brassy notes exploded in perfect time, blending smoothly with Paule's "Island" style music.

The exotic sounds filled the porch with an atmosphere that felt like palm tree visions, and refreshing tropical breezes. The positive vibrations resurrected spirits, like a musical fruit descended from a Bob Marley cultivated legacy.

Oh, but we were just getting started!

Once our musical compulsion ended, I took the liberty to go grab this manuscript. I wanted to share my writing to this point. I was especially anxious for sister Dahli to hear the section that mentions her, in the "Ninja-Mama-Episode."

It was a wonderful impulse. When I read that passage from the manuscript, the words seemed to explode into their ears, exciting their minds, and stimulating the following conversation.

Sister Dahli began by asking: "What does it take to make a man ready for such a responsibility as managing the birth of his own child?"

To this I replied: "Well, first of all, he must "really" believe in, and have close relations with God. His faith has to be strong enough to enable him to receive and carry out "Divine Directives." And, it seems to me that he should also have love, compassion, and empathy in his heart for all people.

Finally, he needs to have knowledge of the Healing Arts, with some Allopathic understanding as well."

Dahli, nearly losing me with her sly, logistical maneuvering, replied: "Well, what about a man who, at 30, 40 or 50 years of age, still "nurses" that tit, running around from tit to tit, sampling and suckling."

I started to answer, but it dawned on me, that, in the not too recent past, I too have enjoyed an occasional good nursing. So, I hedged my answer, retorting: "Well, I was a breast fed baby, and I can still remember my mother's embarrassment, when the mother of a local radio celebrity-who used to live two doors down from our house on Pascagoula Street, between the Funches, and the Andersons—said to me, in front of my mother, . . . "They (the church ladies at Rev. Black's Church-St.Luther) would pass you around, and take turns feeding (nursing) you, even during service."

I smiled, and continued with my attempt to divert the direction of this, now obvious "set-up": "So, I guess I can't totally condemn the "Brothers," of whom you speak." I winked, to let her know that I was aware of the direction of her inference, and of whom she was referring (her "X").

Undaunted by my futile attempt to let her know that she was "busted," she added: "Yes, well, man is a human, yet, he is still an animal . . . an animal who gets nourishment from a mother's breast, just like other animals. If this is not, as you suggest, an indication that the man who keeps on suckling remains in an infantile state of mind, then perhaps it is indication that man may derive some psychological satisfaction, and fulfill some physiological need from the act of "nursing."

Oh, . . . but she-and my wife-were having fun now. I went for their bait, hook, line and attention. That's when they laid it on me.

With a sly grin on the corner of her lip, my wife joined in the fun. Picking up on her "for real soul sister's" lead, she said to me: "So then, it is logical to conclude that, since woman is an human animal as well, could it be that, woman may also need to continue that same act of suckling a breast, feeding, and deriving pleasure, and perhaps some unnamed gratification from the female tit."

Ah, yes, . . . I had fallen into their carefully laid trap, and I thought: "Yeah, and while you are there on that titty, of course other sensuous feelings are aroused, and what the hey, why not just go on and enjoy that (as Grady of "Sanford and Son" put it) "public place," too, and even juicily, and "climaxically" so!"

But, I kept that thought to myself (when I shared this thought with my wife, later, she smiled with a sheepish grin, yet, didn't think it was so funny).

Instead of sharing that thought with the group, I responded by observing: "That's real cute sisters, but tell me this . . ." before I could complete the words of that thought, me and Brother Paule had to "knock on wood," and pinch each other, because he joined in, and we quizzed in two voiced harmony: "Who says that the titty the woman suckles has to be female?"

Still together, we both howled, and jumped up, slapping each other's palms with "high-fives."

Oh, yeah, the men could have some fun too!

But, alas, this little exchange and revelation may have been a bit too much "nasty" talk for our impromptu, yet on-going spiritual session. For, without formally opening or closing the doors of our "home-service," we quickly ended our session. We parted, smiling, bowing, and thanking one another for a much needed communion.

Mamaku and I savored the good feelings our friends brought us, to the end. We followed them to their car, continuing to thank them for bringing us such a glorious Sunday morning.

We returned from the driveway, arm in arm. Mamaku held the baby in her hands, as I danced tenderly, on my bare feet, "hip-hopping" over our front yard, which was worn to dust, by many parked cars, over the past 12 years.

Soon, I didn't have to dance so gingerly, because the dusty ground suddenly started to feel, oh so wonderful. The bottom of my naked feet had become accustomed to the massage of sharp pebbles, and tiny sticks, that lay about the yard. As I reached a certain spot-a long oval shaped indention caused by settling rainwater-I began to feel a wonderful coolness from the deposit left in the not too dried earth. I stopped, and stepped into that cool dry gully, feeling the soothing vibrations of Mother Earth. Just that quickly, another family adventure "was on."

Mamaku sensed my excited discovery, and came back. Facing me, she came in close, touching the tips of her bare toes to mine.

I called for all the children. They came running from the backyard, off the front porch, and from within the house. They immediately picked up on the meaning of our family time discovery. Beaming with joy, they were glad to join in the fun. I instructed Tashi to turn her back to mine, and Rahkua to touch the tips of her bare toes to the tips of Tashi's toes. They did so, and joined hands too, bare feet grounded in the cool earth. Then we told Jolanti to back up to Mamaku, and stand with his back resting gently against his mother's back. Baby Cake (Rah-Imhotep) touched toe tips with 'Lonti, and joined hands as well. He was the only one who displayed any reluctance, but he joined in agreeably, after some coaxing.

We stood there in that spot for a long time, smiling and chattering, while being bathed by warm sunrays, and tantalized by earth's gravitational forces. Oblivious to the Sunday afternoon traffic, and people passing on foot, and watching from nearby porches. We were surrounded and engulfed by good feelings of family love and closeness. The children were thrilled by our reflection, which bounced off the side door of our Mini-van.

We appreciated one another's presence, and we clung together like one big "being," with many legs, and hands, and feet, but with one happy mind and heart.

By now, I bet you are saying: "Yeah, that's nice, but what about the "how-to-birth-your-children-at-home" stuff?

To that question, I say, this sharing of simple pleasure, and expression of love for all family members, is the whole point. This kind of experience satisfies one of our most important criterions of keeping the "expectant mom" in a happy, healthy, and tranquil state. It also provides an opportunity to give much needed attention to those hyper little bodies, and to "chill them out." Calming the children down (some times we do this by "flavoring" their beans with generous amounts of catnip, and Echinacea herb tea), and "cooling them out" reduces stress and strain on Mamaku (not to mention me, as well).

For me, such occasions represent opportunities for spending quality time.

In case we have given the impression that we are all in control, and only do the right thing all the time, let me straighten out that notion.

This Father's Day, beginning so healthily, with breakfast in bed, a card, and gifts of a "waist bag" and computerized watch, with intellectual and spiritually stimulating activities and good times, was destined to end with Mama and Daddy out of control. The following account reveals this fact so very well.

Mamaku walked to the convenience store, a couple of blocks away. She returned with a bag of candy bars, but she hid them until the children were asleep. She insisted later, that I also go to the store. She wanted me to bring back a six-pack of dark beer, and a bag of potato chips. Though I complained briefly, in truth, I was delighted by this naughty turn of events.

So, there we were, ending a glorious day, munching on candy bars, sweets and chocolates, drinking dark beers, and crunching on plain potato chips. Hardly perfect, we now had to concern ourselves with cleaning our bodies of impurities.

Somehow this gorging seems to "cool-Mamaku-out," perhaps because these foods fulfill some nutritional deficiency, or maybe they satisfy some craving needed to satiate a hidden psychological imbalance. (Maybe that's why I grew up fat, eating to solve some human socialization pressure) But, then I'm only speculating. Yet, Mamaku has never consumed this much snack food, at one meal, in any of her previous pregnancies.

I can say, though, she does seem to be happy.

So, you see we are not perfect, even though we try hard to stay on a righteous course, especially when it comes to our diet. Yet, the candy bar craze continued for another day, and it even attracted some cheap red pop.

I could blame this dietary "bust" on Mamaku, and she could blame it on the children. However, regardless of where the fault lies, once we reach our body's tolerance for such onslaughts, sickness is likely to follow. At that point, we must administer the enemas, make the fitting herb teas, give herbal baths, and administer therapeutic massages. At these times, we refresh our body healing understanding by reading and re-reading "Back To Eden:" and other natural healing books, paying close attention to the sections related to the symptoms demonstrated. We also pray for forgiveness for our weaknesses, and for our sickness to be removed.

By the way, during such occasions, some of the important herbs we rely upon to restore balance, and flush out toxins, include: Golden Seal, Comfrey, Echinacea, Catnip, Chickweed, Bayberry Bark, Ginger Root, Slippery Elm, Licorice Root, and Senna Leaves.

As we mentioned, one of the most effective means we employ to restore wellness, involves the use of various forms of massage. Mamaku receives these massages constantly. She's got to have it, and she gets hers every day. In fact, she just rose from the floor, where she had been in Hara (See "Hara," by Karlfried Von Durkheim.). While lying on the floor, she had "gone to her lower belly," with her breath and thought. During the time she was in that meditative state, I had "worked" on her neck, and upper back-which appears to have bowed in exaggeration.

To my pleasant surprise, and unexpected delight, Mamaku felt so good, and was so recharged by the massage ("Body-Reviving-Down-Home-Rub-Down") I gave her, that she felt obliged to do me.

She gave me the most wonderful massage I can remember. I did not realize how badly my own body needed to be touched, and kneaded, "Rolphed," and rubbed with olive oil. Muscles, and whole limbs jerked, stiffened, and relaxed, as deep, unknown pains surfaced and subsided. The more I was stroked, tensions released, and a soothing peaceful calmness rested over my being, until I nearly fell asleep.

Once again, I am not sure, but I think that I may have fallen off to sleep, and started dreaming, yet I could feel my nose flare, and I became aware of myself, when a certain appendage of mine received the attention of the massage. That organ stiffened, and hardened, but unlike the rest of my body, it refused to relax or recoil. The more it was rubbed and stroked, the harder, and more swollen it became. Then, before I knew it, that shining "knight", with a mind of its own, assumed a familiar position astride, and inside its mate-who had been anxiously waiting, throbbing, wide open and juicy. Glad to be together again, the two mates soared on the wings of pleasure. They took an unforgettable journey to ecstasy.

That slow motion journey of unbearable friction, silenced by choice, seemed to last forever. It finally ended in wonderful explosions of joy-releases kept quiet by low moaning lips. Suppressing audible expressions of indescribable sweet feelings, those lips, glued together by the mounting pressure of urgent release, were mindful not to wake the "babes" asleep in the room across the hall.

As you can see, like all the other pregnancies, mother has got to have more than a massage sometimes, . . . that is . . . if I wasn't dreaming.

Days later, when our senses returned, Mamaku felt my concern for our weak, and stumbling constitution, she was acutely aware of our failure to maintain a "straight and narrow" health conscious path. She took steps to change our faltering course. She started by reading to me concerning the virtues of raw food diet, and therapy. She noted that the author-N. W. Walker, D.Sci.-emphasized the importance of fresh raw fruit and vegetable juice. She quoted Walker's theories and propositions that he puts forth in "Raw Vegetable Juices."

She just read a section to me that I must share, but before I do, there is something I have to interject immediately. This concerns a reoccurring state of mind that Mamaku displays, which I have thus far neglected to mention in my notes. I have not recorded this unsettling behavior because I didn't want to give life to the implications of the statements she made concerning the condition of her body.

At first I felt that her refusal to accept the fact that she may be pregnant was merely a reflection of her humorous, and satirical nature working overtime. She would often frown whenever I told a friend that we have been blessed again with the coming of another new life. I also felt that this reaction was due to the fact that she doesn't like to have to deal with those who think she already has too many children, and even go so far as to share their "well meaning" thoughts with her.

As I sit here next to her, on the front porch, with the children settling down inside the house, after a delicious meal, she is reading to me. The latest rejection just passed through her lips. So, I am finally forced to acknowledge this disturbing truth, while listening to her, and writing into this manuscript. She has said all along that she did not know if she were actually pregnant. In the recent past, she quipped: "I don't feel anything down there . . . stop telling folks that. You don't know for sure that I am."

I can no longer ignore this negative reality. I must make note of these comments, and I am beginning to wonder, if I should worry, especially since Mamaku just made a most alarming announcement: "Maybe I've got a tumor."

In the recent past, when my wife made such remarks, I didn't take them too seriously, nor as an indication of denial, because I felt (or wanted to feel) they were made in jest, without strong conviction. However, these incidents are becoming more and more frequent and harder to ignor.

Anyway, we will deal with this situation a little later. Right now, I feel the need to quote Walker's health conscious words that my wife read to me. These words are so very appropriate, particularly as we are confronted with them in the wake of our free wheeling binge on 'junk food."

This particular quote comes from the section in "Raw Vegetable Juices" dealing with Carrot Juice (p.50)

> " . . . . the cleaning of the body by colon
> irrigations and high enemas and by eating sufficient
> volume and variety of fresh raw vegetable juices daily,
> will afford us little or no cause to know from further
> Personal experience what sickness and disease feel like."

This theory of nutritional justification for dietary selectivity is so important for us, because our religious beliefs lead us to conclude that the health of the expectant mom determines her baby's mental and physical qualities, and that mother's personal health and well-being also affect her ability to give birth. The stronger she is, and the better is her physical conditioning, "it stands to reason," and our experiences prove, she has an easier, less painful birthing, especially if she has consumed the proper nutrition.

This is the reason our quest to eat the most healthy food available is greatly influenced by data that describes the highest state of such an art. The next posit, which is quite sobering, we deem from the section in which Dr. Walker deals with Celery Juice. We find this message timely, and very interesting, since it comes on the heels of our over indulgence in the very food he describes (pp. 51-52): In essence he says that raw celery juice is very valuable to people who have been addicted to concentrated sugars all their lives because it contains a high percent of organic sodium and calcium which is needed to repair a system full of concentrated starch and concentrated carbohydrates, including cereals, spaghetti, donuts, ice cream, as well all food products containing processed sugar of any kind. Walker further states that these foods are destructive causes of deficiency that leads to an alarming number of illnesses, because the human digestive system was not meant by Nature to digest and convert this so called food into nourishment; thus the epidemic of degenerative diseases (which presents unsolvable problems for contemporary medical technology) is taking over our bodies almost before adulthood.

If you are like me, the above insight—for which we are grateful to Dr. Walker for sharing—is shocking (even to the degree of "toxic-normality" such as that which we achieve with our own "not too perfect" dietary regimen).

Coincidentally, at this very moment, Mamaku is making a quick move on utilizing this wisdom. As she prepares us more turnip green juice, I am reminded by Dr. Walker of the Calcium and Magnesium depletion caused by Cow's milk (strangely enough, since we've been taught just the opposite all our lives), and the other processed foods about which he says such calcium from animal sources is about as organic as that used to make cement.

For Mamaku this translates into adopting and instituting a religious use of celery, carrot, dandelion, and turnip green (leaf & root) juice to supply her teeth and bones with the strength taken away by our growing embryo.

She just nudged me, and said: "Alleged growing embryo!" Then she got up from her perch next to me, on our porch swing. We had been sharing a Sunday afternoon meal of Collard greens, lima beans, cucumber slices, corn bread, and potato salad (we will talk about this salad later).

I hate to interrupt this discussion of Mamaku's diet, but I must cut in here, with some disturbing news about an "ill-wind" that just blew into our life.

I was coming out of our bedroom, headed for the porch, where everyone except the baby-who was asleep in her crib-gathered for "board games," and a little relaxation, when my wife burst past me, running into the bathroom. She yelled to me: "I feel something wet running down my leg."

To my dismay, she displayed a bloody "show" in her panties. Even though it was small, it caused me some concern, because of the words I had read in "Spiritual Midwifery." This book reveals that it is somewhat normal for a "show" in the early months, . . . but a dark "show" was associated with an aborted pregnancy.

My wife dismissed the possibility. She exclaimed that I had not allowed her to buy a pregnancy test, and that she was still "nursing" Namibiyah, which could explain her missed menstrual cycle. Well I was "not abouts' to fall" into that argument trap. I knew full well that my wife knows very well that she has my support to do as she pleases, when she pleases, . . . and she does. Besides, truth is that, test or no, "visit to a doctor," or not, neither of these actions have the power to cause her "to be or not to be" pregnant.

It does, however, seem that now I do have "pie-in-the-face." Because after that initial dark "show," she produced a redder "show" on her second trip to the "johnette," a few hours later. More than likely, this means that her "Period" has returned. So, now I am red-faced for not having purchased that pregnancy test. But, as we sit here on the floor, in a Yoga position, my wife informs me that it is cheaper to visit a prenatal clinic, than to pay $10 or $15 for a test-which may be found in most grocery stores.

To add weight to her soft argument, after suggesting that I add a chapter to this book that deals with "Complications," she added: "You know that my "Period" came down earlier than usual this time anyway . . . and my teeth were in such bad shape, . . . and, you know we made "Goldberg" too soon, because you couldn't wait any longer, remember?"

Oh yes, I remembered all right. Yet, even though I listened attentively, and thoughtfully to her explanations and rationalizations, my former belief that she was/is pregnant began to regain momentum, and control over my mind set. And, so, as she talks, I'm sitting here thinking: "Yeah, but what about the "Ninja-Mama-Sword¬Swinging-Incident," how do you explain that away?"

Mamaku interrupted my thought, as she continued presenting her "case": "That pregnancy test device never failed me, not since I discovered it four births ago." I replied, half-jokingly: "I know you "did a Tituba" (the reader will have to read the book to know exactly what I am referring to). With a serious look on her face, she replied: "No, I ain't did nothing . . . even though I have been "shooting off," I am a little disappointed myself."

On that note, we suck (I'm going to "mess with the reader's mind now, and see who is concentrating, because that word, suck, is very significant to what has been the subject of jokes about our President (sometimes I think the newscasters and comedians may be a little too disrespectful to the importance of the authority that this office should demand though, in the name of free speech). It made me think about President Clinton, and about the fact that, interjecting that thought AT THIS POINT IN THE MANUSCRIPT, requires explanation, which is that, at this very moment, I am processing my fifth draft of this manuscript, while using a "Lap-Top"-Macintosh, PowerBook 160, thanks to a loan from a family friend, I'm listening to some wonderful Jazz music, on WJSU, while sitting with my wife, on the porch, in the sunshine of a warm and sunny Mississippi "spring-in-the-winter-time" day, on Monday, the first day of March, 1999. So, now, lets return back to the past, when this writing was done.) in our swollen chest, and humbly regroup our dashed hopes, and aborted plans

With no reason to justify any further discussion in this chapter, we bring it to an abrupt close. We also bring closure to our attempt to include a scientific method of data collection into our birthing adventure book.

After we consider the matter of Complications, in our next chapter, we feel obliged to bring our book to a close with our summary chapter. We admit that, disappointment leads us to such a decision. Yet, it is true that we really have covered the essential details that expose our home birth method, and we have shared a good number of birthing stories.

As I get ready to share even more birthing stories, in the final two chapters, my mind is still unable to discount the fact that Mamaku had displayed the pregnancy sign, whereby there is an increase in appetite, and craving for junk food, and odd combinations of tastes, at odd times of the night. And, also, it is hard for me to shake the realization that all those other signs manifested, and I have grown to rely upon them in the past to assure me that Mamaku is "expecting."

Was I that wide of the mark? Or . . . , did she have a miscarriage, for some reason known only to God.

We ponder that question, as we plan the remaining information, which unfolds, not from immediately occurring incidents, but from hindsight revelation, and recollection of pertinent stories that transpired years ago.

CHAPTER 5

COMPLICATIONS

In this chapter we examine the problems we have had to solve, during the use of our Home Birth techniques. We will discuss other incidents similar to the one we just experienced. This will also include problems caused by over work, stress, and strain. Further, we will underscore the role that fear, ignorance, anxious dependence upon "due dates," and other imposed schedules, play in forcing rash choices of action, and justifying potentially harmful procedures. Finally, we elaborate on why we feel that "hurrying the baby along," and such non-medically motivated reasons used to justify dangerous treatments, amount to interference with God's plan of procreation.

First, let us get to that potato salad story I promised . . . , (thought I'd forgotten, didn't you?). By doing so, we may even uncover the cause of the ill-fated complications described at the end of the last chapter.

But, hold on, . . . we have a new development in progress, which demands attention. I am forced to interrupt our efforts to move forward, to halt our flow of thought on the subject of Complications, and set back our attempt to get into the "Amazing Potato Salad Story."

We have sad news concerning Mamaku's condition. It appears that we have proof that my "scientific (if you will)" hunch, observations, and prognosis were correct. It seems that I may have been right about her pregnancy.

She just called me into the bathroom, with a shrill shriek: "Baba . . . come quick!"

When I arrived in the bathroom, almost as quickly as teleportation, she showed me a *clot*, and attempted to convince me that this confirmed her theory. She theorized that her "period" was finally coming down, after having been held up all this time by the healing changes her body had to go through following the delivery of Namibiyah.

Yes, there was a tiny clot in the toilet, however, she also showed me a piece of aluminum foil, which contained a smaller clot, plus a larger, almond shaped mass of tissue covered with blood. The mass was tight, like the inside of a chicken's gizzard. I examined it, as she called me to her side. She was sitting there on the toilet; her face was frozen in a soundless cry. She motioned for me to stand by her, as she held her hands underneath a large piece of tissue that dangled over the water in the toilet bowl. When she finally had a movement, the mass of tissue also fell. She caught it!

What a revelation, the ultimate complication—miscarriage; it seems to be underway even as I write these words. While water runs in the sink, Mamaku quietly yells: "It doesn't hurt anymore!" At least this was encouraging news, because I had begun to worry about her complaints of pain. Only two days ago, she had started complaining of pain in the lower left portion of her belly, but I neglected to record the complaints, because of my disappointment at the prospect that her "period" had come on, and our attempt at being scientific had been thwarted.

But, now she was moved by the power of another kind of pain. She walked nakedly, clad only in house shoes, moving slowly toward my perch on our bedroom easy chair. She held a plastic bag containing the blob of tissue; it looked like a swollen piece of plump beef liver, connected to a thin, light colored rubbery ribbon of lining that looked like chitterling.

How sad! But, we immediately sensed the need to escape the overpowering feeling of depression that attempted to take us over, and hold our minds captive for who knows how long. So, we began to pray. We thanked God for all our blessings, and we asked to be allowed to profit from all our experiences. We resolved that God would not give us more than we can handle, and "goodness knows" we have our hands full.

Though I just acknowledged God's omnipotence, . . . there my mind goes again, trying to find a reason for this alleged miscarriage. So, now I am preoccupied with searching recent events, in hopes of discovering a cause for our mishap. Then, I focus on the memory of the Bar B Q Fish Dinner we just had on our front porch.

Yeah, that was the culprit-that fateful Bar B Q Fish sale. We had finally got around to selling our culinary creations to the community, for the purpose of generating cash to cover our cost of living expenses, while at the same time, testing the market and introducing our delicious vegetarian dishes. I was proud of my tasty Fish-A-Q, and Mamaku's natural good potato salad, which was "dubbed," the "Amazing Potato Salad," by the last visitor of our weekend sale. This sale had been yet another chance to access the market, and attain financial stability and economic viability.

Now, in hindsight, that Bar B Q Fish Dinner Sale seems to have been a grave mistake. It can easily be linked to circumstances that may have caused Mamaku to strain herself. This may have led to an inability on Mamaku's part, to carry our developing embryo to "babyhood."

Mamaku just lay on the bed, after cleaning herself up, in the bathroom. She puckered up for a kiss. With her lips pursed, she asked: "Do you love me Baba?"

Easing back, after planting a little "peck" on her lips, . . . wearing a broad, "happy-to-be-needed" smile on my face, I replied: "You know I love you, honey, . . . now, and always!"

Inside my mind, turmoil turned my quest for reason into a guilt trip. I thought: "I just had to have that Bar B Q Fish venture at this inopportune point in time. After years of dreaming, and pledging to become wealthy by sharing the delicious alternative menus, offering the benefit of years of creating nutritious meals, while substituting for the meat and processed foods, achieving wonderful flavors in the exchange, and showing off our expertise in the use of herbs, spices, fruit and vegetables. Perhaps we were being punished for not being strict vegetarians, who don't even eat so-called seafood. What a time to make a dream come true!"

Actually, I feel even guiltier after further contemplation, because I realize that my wife never really liked the idea of having the sale. She submitted to my plans, bravely pursuing my dream, mainly because she loves to create tasty vegetarian dishes too (She refuses to admit that I introduced her to this art of substituting live, vital and nutritional ingredients into recipes calling for processed, devitalized food, and animal products.)! She must have had a feeling that the physical demands of this "Mom and Pop" business venture might be too much of a burden on her body.

I should have sensed that she was intent on pleasing me, sacrificing her self, always seeming to feel the need to prove to me that she can "make something of herself." Nevertheless, I take refuge in the fact that I am constantly trying to dispel this notion that presupposes condemnation on my part, and indicates a low estimation of self worth.

This apparent lack of confidence, and loss of high self-esteem overtook her mind when she was unlawfully terminated by the Jackson Public School District, for wearing head wraps (according to Judge Fred Banks, the Mississippi Supreme Court, and the U.S. Supreme Court in its silence, this "so-called" "unprofessional attire" could not be viewed as insubordination, and termination on this ground was violation of First Amendment Rights). However, she is yet to receive compensation and redress for this wrong she suffered for exercising her religious beliefs. In fact, she received "double jeopardy violation," as retrial of the same matter, under a claim of "collateral estopel" established "new," erroneous charges, refutable and previously undocumented evidence as grounds for termination: "Dirty-filthy-linty-hair-with-particles-of-lint-in-it;" as previous facts used by Judge Banks in his favorable ruling were not allowed in the retrial!

Undoubtedly, the loss of our alleged embryo exacerbates her recurring bouts with feelings of despair and worthlessness, and having a life of failure-all because of the callous treatment she received that resulted in the termination of a dedicated teacher and single parent, whose ability to provide for her children were thereby ended (Oh, what a shameful act.). So, I have to convince her that she does have worth.

I am no psychiatrist, but I do see the need to constantly reassure my wife that my religious beliefs persuade me to view her ultimate value in terms of a measure of how well she keeps God's word, particularly when it comes to being fruitful and multiplying. I let her know that her commitment to our resolve determines her value and worth to me. I make sure that she knows that I am happy with our "fruit," and proud of her choice to allow our family to grow. However, at this very moment, I must concern myself with convincing her that my love for her is greater than any feelings caused by the possible loss of a child. She must also know that my love is greater still, than her fear that she failed me, because maybe she really just passed a tumor, and was unable to give us another baby, as I had hoped.

Though I feel at fault, I'm not blaming myself or anyone else in the negative sense of the word, because we really did enjoy the Bar B Q sale (does this sound as if I am beginning to lose my mind and "bug-out?" . . . . well . . .).

Looking back on it all, my guess is that this alleged miscarriage happened as result of the enormous amount of energy we had to expend in order to get our house and business in order. We had to complete tasks that had gone undone for years. This had to be taken care of before we were ready to handle all the tasks involved in introducing our healing food mission, which we view as part of our overriding purpose. We see a direct correlation between this unsuccessful attempt to begin providing our community with a source of wholesome vegetarian and macrobiotic cuisine, and our Alternative Naturopathic Healing Mission.

It is our belief that God wants us to serve our community as Healing Agents, involved as Healthy Life Style consultants, Home Birth Advocates, Health Food and Vegetarian Diet Counselors, and Spiritual Massage Servants. Yet we find ourselves in a dilemma. We wanted to market the products of our forty "some odd years" of combined experience as students of the Healing Arts, but we find no significant financial support, nor do we possess the energy to continue writing proposals, and constantly promote Health Programs and products we have received through prayer, meditation, and experimentation; including, Mamaku's Orange Sunshine-a pain relief salve, and Dr. Daddy's Herb Sacks-various herbal blends to solve common ailments.

Of course, we must always "work" on ourselves, because fighting illness is a "never ending" job, so we still manage to keep this Healing Service dream alive. Yet, sometimes we are not strong enough to maintain strict observance of the "Principles Of Healthy Living" (see Appendix D), which we developed during our deepest period of commitment to health issues. But, we need the support, and strength of "like minded" people, working on wellness goals, aimed at healing our community and nation.

The above contemplations lifted our spirits, and, since we had "run low" in our supply of fresh herbs, we decided to visit the Health Food Store, where we were sure to find a source of people with healing ideals. For, not only did we need to replenish our supply of herbs and organically grown foods devoid of preservatives and chemicals, but we also needed to commune with people who believe as we do.

Were we in for a treat, and a lift for our battered spirits, just the thing to revive a failed desire to complete this literary project, we call: "Adventures In Home Birthing."

We went to the Rainbow Health Food Store, driving my brother Sam's Maxima, which I had borrowed for a weekend trip to Epps, Alabama, where Mamaku was scheduled to participate as a Story Teller in a Festival put on by the Farm Cooperative. I decided to remain outside the store, in the car with "all my young-uns," pun intended. I figured that was the only way Mamaku could shop in peace.

As I sat there, playing with baby Namibiyah, and attempting to placate the tormenting screams coming from our thwarted little store wreckers, who could not believe they were not going to get the opportunity to terrorize the herb bends, fruit display and drink coolers, I was pleasantly surprised by the sound of a sweet and familiar voice. I turned to see that Blue had taken time from her busy schedule to come out to speak to us.

Blue-one of the founders of our health food store connection here in Jackson, Mississippi, asked me where I'd been for so long. I responded cheerfully: "I haven't been doing too much . . . , just being "House Dad," and writing a book on how we birth our children at home." She perked up with a smile, as her interest peaked. I continued: "However, I have developed a bad case of "writer's block," my stream of grammatical consciousness and thought flow has come to a halt. I'm no longer enthused by the stories of our child birth experiences." With an empathetic look on her face, Blue quizzed: "Why?" I replied: "Well, I "kinda" feel that no one will take too much stock in what I have to say, since I think that maybe we just lost a child . . . Oh, that's right, you didn't know that Akua was pregnant again."

Blue had been hanging on my every word. When I finished, she responded thoughtfully, with sympathetic and sensitive eyes, which beamed from her bright sunshiny smile. She encouraged me with the following reassuring words: "No, RahLeeCoh, please don't feel that way, because what you all just experienced is part of your total picture, . . . your learning about

71

the birth process, and the phenomenon of procreation. What happened to "yall" can, and does happen many times over, even in the hospital, where they may be better prepared and equipped to handle emergency situations. There may be countless number of untold reasons why you all may have lost a child. Perhaps God was letting Akua know that her body-still in the "baby nursing" mode-would not be strong enough to carry the baby safely. RahLeeCoh please don't despair, finish your writing, because we need the kind of sensitive in-depth analysis that I am sure you offer, " . . . and, we would love to carry your book in the store."

With those words of encouragement, and confiding faith, I received renewed inspiration to get back to writing this book. What a wonderful and healing trip to the Health Food Store was this; not only did we obtain healing sustenance for our bodies, we were also blessed with inspiration for our mind and soul, as well.

Appreciative for having my "writer's block" removed, all I can think of is: "Thank God for Blue!"

Now that the flow of words has commenced, my mind keeps telling me that my wife was in fact pregnant. However, I have conceived another theory for the reason the miscarriage occurred. I believe that she got too involved with the book, "I Tituba, Black Witch of Salem," as did I. I think she got so involved; she identified too deeply with Tituba's torment, and unfulfilled suffering. Then she (Mamaku) created a less painful ending to Tituba's story; she wanted to make sure that Tituba got the child she wanted so much. (I know I run the risk of delving into spiritual and supernatural speculation, but tell that to my heart, and the thoughts flowing through my mind.) So, I can visualize an image of Mamaku's super-subconscious mind, unselfishly sending the spirit of our unborn child to Tituba. In Mamaku's Epilogue (if you will), she named this child "Rah¬Healyah." This name suggests a God sent baby girl, who has the power to mend Tituba's persecuted soul.

Mamaku's love for people, particularly persecuted and unjustly treated persons, is so sincere that she gives of herself to them, freely and even naively sometimes.

Though we ponder this question of a possible aborted pregnancy, and the reasons why, we are, nevertheless, still bathed by the memory or Blue's inspiring words. So, as we resume our daily notation form of recording observations, and dealing with the nature of the complications we've experienced, we offer one last story to settle this matter of miscarriage.

Our story begins after a family trip to the library. We made it there and back safely, in our little '85 Escort, which my children playfully call our "Hoopty." They call it this because it is easily the "raggediest" vehicle on the road, with its dusty black, Henry Ford color, accented by a cracked windshield-which was the only glass in that dented body, whose bare parking light bulbs bore witness to many "push starts." I am blessed to have children who appreciate the simple things in life. Instead of being embarrassed by our "ride," their pretty little faces were all smiles, as they "egged" their Daddy on: "Go Daddy . . . , Go Daddy." They sang in unison, as their heads popped up and down, in and out of the glassless side windows and back hatch. Mamaku is "Heaven sent" too, because she gets a kick out of climbing through the windows, and "popping" that stick shift, as we "fly" down the street. We can move so fast because the engine is a "nother" matter entirely. Unlike the body the engine runs perfectly, because "Baba" keeps it tuned, so we can zip in and out of traffic quickly and smoothly, driving defensively to avoid the big cars that give a contemptuous bumper to little old cars.

This library trip is not our regular, every Thursday library visit-when Mamaku checks out about twenty colorful and exciting books, that we take turns reading to our children, and to one another. We made this trip so that our resident family "dramatic art star," Rahkua, could register for a talent show, as a singer. She has won awards for her Harriet Tubman portrayal, at Jackson State, and performed this same act, and other cultural arts sketches in programs hosted by the sweet little old ladies at the Smith Robinson Senior Citizen Center-where I taught classes in "Color Healing and Painting Therapy."

At the audition, Rahkua realized what her mother and I already knew, which is that, true enough, she is prepared to recite Mari Evans, Langston Hughes, Helen Steiner Rice, Shelia Hamanaka, James Weldon Johnson, Henry Dumas, and her mentor-Eloise Greenfield, but she really had not put that kind of time into perfecting any particular song (she wanted to be a singer without "paying her dues"). So she decided not to register.

Back home, sitting at the kitchen table talking to my wife, as she prepares Red Beans and Brown Rice, I read the last entry into this book. Upon hearing how Blue responded, Mamaku threw a new monkey wrench into our "Complications" wrinkle, and my "guilt trip" dilemma. She said: "You know, it could have been the caffeine. I just read somewhere that caffeine may possibly cause miscarriage . . ." In disbelief, I said: "What . . . I thought you said . . . ."

Before I could finish my statement, she cut me off, and added: "You know, I began drinking coffee early on, every morning at the Day Care where I worked. It was sort of a half hearted attempt to ease the pressure of administrative insensitivity, and the demanding needs of the children. But, I guess I was really just giving in to a habitual temptation started and ended many years ago, when I worked in the Public School System."

When I heard the above announcement, I decided right then and there, to put an end to all speculations about what happened, and why we won't be having a child "this time around."

I made up my mind to seek positive meaning, and to find the self-improvement message in this miscarriage experience. We pray for the strength to be able to stick even closer to the Health Teachings that God has allowed us to discover and follow. This has been our "insurance;" it has enabled Mamaku to stay in shape, and bring forth viable and healthy new life.

With that sobering thought, we start and finish by embracing and clinging tighter to our practice of herbal use, vowing to get even more strict in keeping our diet on the mark of vital food intake and harmful food avoidance.

As we make our silent pledge, Mamaku is preparing Pennyroyal-Cayenne-Echinacea Herb Tea; it will help her body to eliminate the remaining clot and tissue fragments. I am drinking ice cold Sassafras, and Ginger Water, plotting my way out of this chapter on Complications.

Although the traumatic events of this chapter caused a drastic alteration in our plans, we are ready to summarize on the nature of complications that we have encountered in our birthing experiences. Accordingly, we see the need for being prepared to prevent or remedy the following situations. First, it is essential that the expectant parents understand the course of action needed to solve the problem one faces, when the umbilical cord is wrapped around the baby's neck. It is true that hindsight paints a picture of a really simple, and natural course of action, but the sight is quite alarming. The key is not to panic, and to remain cool, avoiding decision making motivated by fear.

Secondly, there was the late delivery of the placenta. We've heard some horrible stories of how this can be a life and death situation for the "delivering mother." For us, it seems that fear and lack of knowledge (and failure to act, using information already learned from reading) played a negative role. Not knowing what to do, and being uncertain and fearful, may have led us to make unsound, and unwise decisions. Yet, according to our Traditional Healer friend and teacher, there is no need for worry about the placenta, because women in Africa, who have their babies naturally, as we choose to do, have been known to retain the placenta in their bodies long past the time frame that caused us to fret. They operate on the axiom stating that "the placenta always delivers." Be that as it may, after that frightening situation, regardless of whether or not our fears were groundless, we make sure that Mamaku has plenty of Penny royal herb tea to drink, while she waits for the placenta to deliver. (It appears that the danger comes in to play, if rough hands sever the tissue from the walls of the womb, breaking blood vessels, and causing internal hemorrhaging.) We base this precautionary measure on the claim found in "Back To Eden," whereby Pennyroyal is supposed to have the power to promote delivery of the placenta.

Next, there was the miscarriage-the ultimate complication. We've already discussed several factors that could have been responsible for such a loss, including physical strain, poor diet, and possibly even mental and spiritual drain. For my wife, the solution to this awful consequence lies in a renewed effort to regain former discipline, taking care to avoid all potentially harmful lifestyle choices, including no smoking, and no alcohol or other "hard" drinks (including soft drinks).

Finally, we have mentioned the role that fear can play in magnifying feelings of despair, and lead to desperate courses of action. The following story serves as an example of how fear can actually lead to complications, by influencing decisions that have negative consequences. In this case, though it was not the only culprit, fear influenced two friends of ours into making decisions, we feel, resulted in the justification for a C-Section delivery. They made an unsuccessful attempt to deliver their own child at home. I believe they failed because of several reasons: 1.) their birthing room did not meet the requirements we noted in Chapter 3; 2.) difference of opinion regarding natural birth, opposing religious and cultural beliefs, and disapproving attitudes about home childbirth created an atmosphere full of disharmony, unrest, and tension; 3.) the "expectant father" did not have control over the birthing situation; and 4.) the "expectant parents" faith in God was not strong enough to overcome the fear and uncertainty surrounding the delivery time frame, the unsuitable conditions, and the intense pain that the "first time expectant mother" experienced.

As this was their first child, perhaps inexperience, and doubt caused by fear of the unknown shook their faith. Whatever the reasons, as the story will reveal, the obstacles they faced in their first attempt at home birth proved to be too great for their efforts. (We are happy to report that their second attempt was successful, yet not without the complication of internal hemorrhage, which we have prayed not to have to deal with, even though we have prepared for such a possibility, through research, and by stocking a supply of Cayenne, and Alum.)

And so another story goes:

We pulled into our driveway, exhausted by our return trip from Meridian, MS. The ninety-minute trip took about three hours, because we had plenty of trouble on the road. The trouble was not with the Engine I rebuilt just before the trip, nor was it caused by failure of the CV Joint, and the Spindle and Hub I replaced. It seemed to stem from a mysterious "electrical short" that appeared after a mechanic "friend" of mine helped me install an alternator.

The changes me, and my wife went through because of this trouble, left us physically drained. We had to drive down the highway with dim lights, and a battery that continued to have a power drain or "electrical short," which meant that we had to make many stops to get "boosted off" and to recharge the battery. In addition, our burden was even heavier because of the emotionally taxing experience we encountered when we reached Meridian to find Mamaku's mother critically ill. Since our religious beliefs, and medical practices diametrically oppose the "Intensive Care" treatment she was receiving, we felt a kind of tiredness that was deep and consuming.

All those thoughts, and tribulations weighed heavily on my mind and body, as I pulled into our driveway. When we got closer to the house, I spotted a note sticking out of our screen door. The note contained a frantic message:

> Zim is in "Labor," I've gone
> to buy some water. We need
> you all to come over and
> deliver our baby.
>
> Sal, 9:00PM

By the time we read the note, it was around 11:OOPM Sunday night. We were already too tired, but, after we finished unpacking, and carrying in our sleeping "fruit," we were, without a doubt, famished.

Shortly, the anticipated knock at the door caught us unsettled and unprepared. It was Sal all right. He was in an excited haste, and he wanted us to come with him.

My wife and I decided that it would be best if she went alone, and I could relieve her in a little while. Unfortunately, when I was ready to leave, I discovered that Mamaku had inadvertently taken the keys to the van, so I couldn't leave. This was probably just as well, though, for, I would have had to leave our children "home alone," during the period of time it would have taken for me to drive over to Sal's and back with Mamaku, before I could return to Sal's to assist Zim. Unless, of course, Mamaku drove back alone, leaving me there, that would still have been a good bit of time to leave our babies alone.

By now, our home was dark and silent, as all the little noisemakers were silently "calling the hogs, and counting sheep." Though I was anxious about being unable to leave, time moved swiftly, through periods of restlessness, and indecisiveness about whether or not to go to sleep. I had the feeling that, if I went to sleep, since my body and mind were so stressed out, it would be impossible for Mamaku to awaken me. Before I knew it, the clock showed the time to be, 7:30AM.

It was then, that Mamaku finally returned home. She was really worn out, agitated and frustrated. Though she was uneasy, and in need of releasing her frustration story upon my ears, she did not have time to talk, because her "ride" would return for her, in a few hours. She did take time to tell me that Sal's house was in a state of frenzy, and they were worried out of their minds, over the fact that Zim's water bag had burst, and the signs of delivery readiness were lagging behind what everybody expected, except Mamaku, who felt that they were unnecessarily concerned, and alarmed falsely. She based her opinion on her own experience, which led her to believe, that, although the labor seemed to be lasting a long time, the baby really was not yet ready to come forth. Further, she felt that since this was Zim's first birth, labor could be expected to last a lot longer than it would normally. Mamaku told me that she tried unsuccessfully to get this point over to a house full of too many people (mother and sister of the "expectant dad," sister and best friend of the "expectant mom") divided by opposing political, religious, and social views and affiliations. So, it was no wonder that she looked haggled and weary. She had just left a birthing situation full of doubt and fear, and too many minds that really disapproved of natural birthing at home, or any naturopathic assistance my wife was prepared to offer, and agreed to provide (as it turned out, for free). The climate created by these friends and relatives of this stressed couple who needed a certain kind of compassionate culturally oriented birthing relief, caused a hopeless and somber mood to settle over the atmosphere in that "would be" home birth situation. This troubled mood followed Mamaku home, reflecting itself in her exhausted spirit.

After taking a bath, and nodding off for a couple of hours, Mamaku revived soon enough to be picked-up by Zim's "friend girl." They returned to the "scene of the birthing."

Mamaku did not return home until about 7:00PM, the next evening. She was in terrible shape. Mentally, and physically she was "spent," and wrenched. The experience of having to deal with her critically ill mother, and leaving, only to run into a situation that was even more stressful and draining, was a bit too much for Mamaku, especially when you consider the fact that she was also pregnant.

Before she fell into deep sleep, she told me that Zim had been calling for me to come, and deliver her baby. Through her drooping eyelids, and between gasping yawns, she went on to let me know also, that everyone in the house, except herself, still believed that the baby was overdue. She continued by slipping in a sad note; she said that Zim had been asking for me, and felt that I did not love her, since I had not come to help them deliver her child. Trailing off with a husky groan, Mamaku barely finished by whispering that Sal's mother was there, and she was definitely opposed to home birthing.

As she ended in a loud snore, before finishing that last whisper, she added in the same breath that Zim's sister was also there, but had a more accepting and permissive attitude.

All kinds of crazy thoughts raced through my mind; like, I am not legally protected nor authorized to deliver someone-else's baby, and how would Sal feel later, when he realize that I don't have a medical degree and I have "seen" his wife. What kind of a strain would that put on our friendship?

It was at that point that I decided to go into "Hara," and to meditate, seeking "Divine Counsel, and direction from God, as to what should be my course of action.

I remained in the 5th position of Hara (see Karlfried Von Durkheim), on my knees, with my buttocks resting on, and cradled by my ankles, while my palms were facing upward, resting gently on my thighs for quite a while.

I received messages and visions. I sought to make spiritual contact with Zim and her unborn child. I made contact; it was a kind of "sub-reality perception connection." I COULD ACTUALLY FEEL THE TENSION IN THE BIRTHING ROOM. I sensed uneasiness from the baby, and hysteria from Zim. I received the revelation that Zim needed to be calmed down, the baby needed to be coaxed and reassured, and that Sal had to take control of the situation, and bring peace into the birthing room. I even received a name for the baby (Ironically, or coincidently enough, this name-Saleem, was very similar in sound and close to the name actually chosen by Sal and Zim, as I discovered sometime later.); they named him Salim.

I felt the urge to put the principles and practice of Psychic Healing to work in order to allow myself to improve the situation (I reveal this secret art to you in strict confidence, because Benjamin 0. Bibb, and Robert J. Weed, in "Psychic Healing;" warn against telling people that you practice this art. They say you should be silent about its use.). Following the procedural steps they outline for putting this powerful technique to work, I proceeded to put my imagination, and subconscious mind to the task of contacting the "ethereal-selves" of both mother and child.

In that state of mental-spiritual awareness, I was able to explain to Kim that I really did love her, and that I would help (Of course, I could only do this after creating an imaginary skit, whereby an operator reached Zim's subconscious mind, after instructions from me, whereupon I received permission to proceed. See "Psychic Healing" for detailed instructions). I continued by telling her that she should calm down, not panic, and trust in God. Then, I let Saleem—as I had envisioned his name to be—know that, even though the atmosphere outside of his mother's womb was filled with chaos and misunderstanding, he could come out anyway because everybody loved him, wanted to meet him, and needed him to come out now, especially his mother.

After I was done communicating with mom and babe through imagination, and metaphysically, I initiated contact with dad (Sal), whom I advised of the exhausting situation we just underwent in Meridian, and on the road between Jackson, on the way back. I also explained to him about the importance of harmony and peace, and, order and cleanliness in the birthing room, and home, before I concluded this purpose filled meditative state.

When I finally left home, I was confident about my spiritual directive. I was also reassured by Mamaku's medical assessment of the birthing situation. As far as she was concerned, the baby was more than likely, on schedule, and, the notion of an overdue, and prolonged labor existed only in the anxious minds that were "under the influence" of fear. As I got nearer and nearer to Sal and Zim's house, I made up my mind. I was not going to deliver their baby. However, I decided that I would assist Sal, guiding him by explaining the steps and procedures that we follow with our own children's births.

As I approached their house, I could see that it was very dark and deserted. The lonely blackness beamed through the shiny pane in their screen door, like a bright opaque light. Through that weatherizing outer portal, I couldn't help but observe that the entry door was left open, an unmistakable sign-testimony of a troubled flight.

I was immediately filled with disappointment, yet, consumed by feelings of relief, and "lost limbo land let down," while my soul was simultaneously stirred with indecisive yearning. I did not know where to go or what to do.

The over powering urge to get to safety took over my will, and ended the state of momentary immobility and uncertainty, into which I had begun to slip deeper and deeper. So, I quickly returned home, as guilt and doubt did battle in my mind, and wrecked havoc on my emotions.

Once I reached the shelter of home, I did not know what to do with myself. I felt guilty about not rushing right over, as soon as Akua told me that Zim was calling for me. I knew that they did not want to go to the Hospital. I guessed they did so, as a last resort. This must have hurt, because they were kindred spirits; and, like us, they too pursued a holistic way of life (in some ways to a greater extent than we do).

I thought: "Oh, what they must think of me, . . . they had to pass right by our house, on the way to the hospital (the same way my Brother Sam had done, five years previous, as he took our Mama on her last trip to the Hospital against my wishes and knowledge)." I wondered if this occurred while I was praying and meditating.

As we come to the "point" of this story, I discovered from Sal, a few days later, that their baby was a boy, and he was brought into this world as result of that dreaded complication referred to as C-Section.

This procedure, as well as Allopathic treatment in general, was not in agreement with their religious beliefs, nor their Naturopathic studies. There is no wonder that Zim appeared to be left with a deep emotional scar immediately after. Her conversations reveal evidence of pain and a long-standing period of mourning over having submitted to a compromise of their beliefs.

Sal also informed me that he had to remove his wife and son from the hospital by force. He claimed that the treatment Zim received there caused her to become sicker, and sicker, and there was even talk of an operation. This possibility and threat upset Sal and he seemed to feel that, since they are a "mixed racial couple," and he is a Dredlock Brother in Mississippi making a family, she was the target of a conspiracy to eliminate such marriages. All he needed was to see his wife growing weaker, to convince him to snatch his family up, and "bust" them out of that hospital. (As of the date of this entry, a couple of years later, they are doing fine, Mother is healthy, and strong, and their second attempt at home birthing, blessed them with a pretty little fat baby girl.)

Some may disagree, but for me the foregoing story illustrates my contention that fear and the pressure caused by allowing "due date hype" to determine course of action leads to negative consequences and complications such as having the baby cut out of mother's womb. This story also presents a prime example of how discord, disagreement about appropriate medical procedures, and the resulting doubt can lead to a loss of faith and confusion. This makes the "delivering mom's" job much more difficult, and as we've seen, may lead to choices that can end in a C-Section (we offer a profound judgment about this procedure in then next chapter.)

This story also underscores the role that **pain** can play in causing decision-making that leads to complications. I reach this determination after that last conversation with Zim. When I told Zim that I had gone into deep meditation, and communicated with her and her son, I asked her if she felt anything, or received a mental message from me at any point. She replied: "The only message that I could hear that night was the piercing sound of pain that pounded me senseless, and drove me out of my head."

On that painful note, we end our consideration of the kind of complications for which our experiences indicate the prospective parents should prepare. With this understanding, we are ready to summarize on the whole process of home birthing we follow when we deliver our children at home.

CHAPTER 6

SUMMARY OF ISHAKARAH HOME CHILDBIRTH TECHNIQUES

AND

BIRTHING EXPERIENCES

In this chapter we will make a quick dry run," and look at the total process involved in our approach to having children-making babies, and giving birth to them at home. Focusing on the important points that lead to a successful delivery, we intend to limit our birthing stories, as we expose certain accepted contemporary medical practices relating to childbirth. In doing so, while praying that we are not lynced, we "step out on a limb" by condemning such procedures which appear to have no basis in science, and may even have grave consequences for the expectant mother and unborn child. In particular, we take a critical look at the connection between the "water bag breaking procedure," and the high incidence of C-Section births. We begin the summary of our childbirth procedures by noting the importance of maintaining close contact with God for spiritual power and Divine revelation and direction.

Throughout this challenging work, we have continuously promoted the belief that guides our procreation efforts-faith in God is the essential ingredient in the home childbirth equation. It allows the prospective parents to gain the knowledge of the natural birth process, as well as some understanding of the prevailing Allopathic medical theories concerning childbirth. This necessary and indispensable element of faith also provides the courage and strength to meet the requirements and accomplish the steps to obtain a successful outcome. With God's help, one is ready to accept this challenge and "stay the course," faithfully seeking knowledge on the birth process. This ultimately leads to consultation with experts in the field, including Mothers, Fathers, Physicians, Midwives, Herbalists, Nurses, and Healers. This conscientious path also leads to knowledge gained as result of contact with the appropriate literature, and association with like-minded individuals.

Obviously, it is very important for one to seek and receive as much knowledge as possible on the subject of birthing before embarking on such a journey (There is nothing like "hands on" experience, though, to clear up the fuzzy pictures created in your mind by all the different views, advice and instructions you get about what to do, and what to expect.) Equipped with the wisdom, and knowledge gained from research and consultation, Dad is ready to help Mom prepare for her ultimate task, provided, of course, that the pregnancy signs discussed in the Introduction, and in Chapter 2, manifest themselves.

Preparation for home childbirth includes a health conscious dietary regimen that considers, and provides for the growing and nurturing needs of both Mother and Child. It helps immensely, if the whole family practices these eating, drinking, and nutriment consumption habits and practices, as a matter of everyday course of action. For us, this means eating foods (for the most part) that are live and vital; and supplementing this diet with choice herbs, fresh squeezed juice, the purest water available, and a pregnancy blend of vitamins and minerals.

To prepare the Expectant Mother for her task, we see that it is necessary for her body and mind to be loved, well conditioned, tuned and exercised as well. In my wife's case, this is achieved through long daily walks, regular massages, positive conversations with empathetic and sympathetic minds, and by maintaining a scheduled plan of exercise, including stretching and bending such as that offered in "Positive Pregnancy Fitness." And, most importantly she needs to be constantly reassured of her beauty, and her desirability; the "Expectant Dad" must demonstrate his love, and convince her that her pregnancy is a blessing from God.

Preparation and readiness for conducting new life into existence must also include establishing and maintaining a clean, safe, peaceful and sanitized environment, which is stocked with the tools and materials needed for delivery. This translates into completing a checklist that includes establishing a birth room, ordering family and business responsibilities, stocking food and supplies-such as sterile blades and clamps to secure the umbilical cord, towels, sheets, and acquiring things, that may or may not be needed, but provide mental security (See Chapter 3).

An assured and confident state of mind comes with knowledge and wisdom gained from a good supply of reference materials. This kind of confidence and peace of mind is invaluable in making this goal an achievable reality. These books and journals should answer questions by providing examples of birthing stories, pregnancy fitness guidelines, and healing art remedies, and solutions for common problems that may be encountered. They are especially helpful in the event of complications or altered plans, at which time, communication with God is more essential than ever to obtain the strength and guidance needed to pull off this event of a life time.

It should be very clear by now, that mastering this awesome responsibility requires that both "expecting parents" must overcome the "fear factor." If your experience is anything like ours, your mind will be filled with a thousand fears, mostly of horrible things that could happen at any stage of this life perpetuating process. However, it is of utmost importance to keep a "cool head." Do not panic! Trust in God makes this possible for Dad. Mom must have a "working belief' in God, as well as faith in Dad's abilities. This gives her strength to withstand pain, and overcome fear.

I cannot say enough to express how good I feel about my wife's bravery, and the confidence she places in me, when she allows me to assist her. Any expectant mom who allows her mate this freedom, and gives him permission to undertake such a feat deserves the utmost praise throughout the entire adventure in home birthing, especially from the appreciative expectant dad.

The expectant Dad's abilities and merit are put to task further (those words "put to," just reminded me of a conversation I had with an African brother from the Continent, wherein he informed me that the term for the pregnant mom about to deliver is: "put to bed"), as he is charged with the important responsibility of making sure that his mate remains in a calm and positive state of mind. There are several things that he can do to keep her in good spirits, and feeling good about their shared commitment. He should make sure that the birthing environ is filled with love, peace, sweet healing smells, soothing lighting, and relaxing sounds. He can also help her stay in a healthy happy state, as we have continuously stressed, by giving her undivided attention, particularly in the form of "Olive oil Massages." He can keep her happier still, by "rapping" and "sweet talking" to her, and by providing her with plenty of fresh fruit and vegetables, vitamin supplementation, along with an ample supply of herb tea (in our case, this means stocking, preparing and serving our own "Pregnancy Blend" of several important herbs; see Chapter 2

The thought of how important herb tea is to our "Birthing Rituals" (if you will), reminds me of the story about the birth of our daughter-Rahkua (and this is the last story, I promise).

As I can remember, at the time of this story, my wife was not yet sold on the idea of us having our babies at home (even though we had Tashi in the back seat of Tiny's Cab), so I had to go along with her wish to use the so called "Natural Birth Wing" of a local hospital. She was persuaded to use this facility because a long time family friend was a doctor on staff at that hospital. This friend agreed to arrange for my wife to be admitted under her care, and to deliver our child.

We were excited by this prospect, and thankful to have such good friends, and such a blessing. So, when we reached the hospital, we were very happy, and in a good mood. We had waited, according to my wife's instructions, until the contractions were about five minutes apart. Mamaku's experience as a four-time mother caused her to be confident and glad to have the support of me and our oldest daughter-Estinika, as we made our way blindly into a medical situation we naively assumed shared our definition of "Natural."

After signing Mamaku "in," we wheeled her to the birthing room, as she "nursed" a cup of her favorite herbal blend-Red Raspberry and Squaw Vine, flavored with a little Valerian Root (added for its nerve calming effect)herb tea. We approached the natural birth room like joyful lambs, full of great expectations.

That joyous exuberance ended abruptly, and our feelings changed. In an instant, the smiles faded from our unbelieving lips, as two nurses, who were not very charming, greeted us. Actually, we were not really greeted by them; they "sorta" ordered, and motioned us in, by the force of these words: "Oh, . . . you can't drink that in here!"

We knew then, that we were "in for it." Upon entering that cold and "unnatural" room, the above admonition rattled, and echoed off unfriendly images of clinical materialism pretending to be "straight and natural", and ready to do battle with our need for spiritual grounding, and divine sanctification for our commitment to be fruitful.

Feeling that things could, and would get worse, our thoughts were confirmed, as those two disagreeable attending nurses "eyed" us contemptuously. As quickly as they grunted out responses to our curiosity, they spread some black "gook" on both sides of Mamaku's swollen belly. Then, just as quickly, even before an objection could leave our lips, they attached two clumbsy electrical devises to her belly. Our protests were met with a snobbish authoritative air, and a condescending "ig"-aware of its power and legal protection, followed by a pretentious grunt that would have us believe it was all done to protect and monitor the baby.

Mamaku-adorned by a serenely brave and reverent smile, seemed to rest unwarily, oblivious to my vision of her as the "sacrificial offering" to this unnatural trickery. She was regal in her acceptance of the fate for which we had brought ourselves to this contemporary alter. The shocking reality of how different our view of natural birth is from what was being imposed upon us, and the vision of my wife lying there on that paper sheet bedding caused my mind to flash back to when I WAS FACED WITH THIS SAME KIND OF A DILEMMA, AT A CRUCIAL POINT IN MY MOTHER'S HOSPITALIZATION. Like now, I disagreed then, with the type of treatment she was (my mother) receiving. I felt then, as I do now-helpless! I envisioned police, and handcuffs, straight jackets, and jail cells as official response to my objections, to my rage, and the urge to pick my mother up and run out of there. But, it really was too late anyway. I had warned, and pleaded with her; I BEGGED HER NOT TO GO BACK INTO THAT HOSPITAL. I ASKED HER TO USE THE FAITH SHE AND MY FATHER INSTILLED IN ME . . . , WAIT ON GOD, AND "THE HERBS OF THE FIELD." Yet, she came back-in largely because certain members of our family took it upon themselves to prove to me, as they put it, that: "Those bananas and celery, and "thangs" don't work, you better let that girl go back into that hospital." While I was arrested and taken out of my mother's house, in hand cuffs, falsely accused of trespassing, she was admitted, and a hole was "sawed" into her skull to remove a tumor that, according to the PDR, resulted from the Dilantin she took, which was prescribed by the very same doctors who butchered her head and brain. So, there she was, my Mama, lying on that hospital bed, with the right side of her head shaved, and black bowtie stitches making an oval shaped ring around her swollen scalp. With puffed, half shut eyes, she pleaded with me to take her out of there, yelling hysterically: "They gone hurt me, "git" me out of here! You know I didn't want to come back into this place!"

Broken hearted at this terrible sight, I turned to leave, replying: "They've already done it Mama." With my head hanging down, I left without doing anything. I tried to relieve my guilty feelings by telling myself that I had tried to get her off the pork, all the other animal products, and chemically processed food for years. I had also warned her about those so-called drug "side effects" (I call them "front effects"). None of this conversation with myself made me feel that I was any less guilty. In fact, eventually I had to face the fact that she sacrificed herself to save me; she knew the predicament I was in, opposed by family members who disagreed with my medical position. (I truly believed and still do, that her condition could be remedied by God's herbs and Alternative Healing Systems, even the Brain Tumor, that the Doctor's caused through their prescription of Dilantin, yet, claimed they "misdiagnosed"— even without blame or accountability for her pain and suffering and shortened life). But this kind of therapy is not a "quick fix," you have to be willing to wait, as you apply the remedies, according to Ehret and Gregory, sometimes for as long as it took to get sick. I am convinced that my mother wanted to protect me from a confrontation with Emergency Medical Personnel, who might provoke my rage, during those tense moments, when she was wrestled from my care. I'm sure she thought that hospital emergency would end like all the other ones; but it did not. She paid a "dear" price!

Well here it was again, another "loved one" needed me to rescue them (she is the closest to my heart, now that inappropriate medical treatment caused my Mama to die ten years ago). "It is a little different this time,"-I thought, watching my wife lying in a similar state of helplessness—"at least this time I wont leave, and I'll be here to watch over her." I attempted to comfort my wife, massaging her, and "cooing" her, conscious of the disapproving cold stares emanating from those two disagreeable nurses.

Even though I "busied" myself attentively reassuring Mamaku, I really felt "null and void," and I feared the worst. (I thought about my mother again; she seemed to always expect the worst, and then accept whatever was the actual outcome. I always aim at being positive, but quite naturally, I am influenced by this predilection of my Mother's own response to life stimuli.) So it is no wonder that I felt the ulterior plan was to condition us to accept C-Section birth-what they had in mind all along for our unborn baby, even if it was for no other reason than to make sure that we conform to the norm, or if it were simply maintenance of a continuum of blind procedural policy adherence.

Thinking of the notion of "worst possible scenarios," my mind drifted to the story Mendelsohn (in "MALe Practice") tells of Anarca-the young slave woman who was brutally experimented upon, by Marion J. Simms. For his "inhuman-opium drugging¬Vesi-Covaginal Fistula-butchery," he received a Nobel Prize. This, according to Robert S. Mendelsohn, is one of the many ways that the male dominated medical system humiliates women, and "keeps them in their place." For me, the point revolved around the same issue, the belief system. This includes the norms and values and biases and prejudices, of who ever administers the medical treatment, in addition to their choice of methodology, and medical practice which is based on certain assumptions, and theoretical justifications for prognosis and prescription. Thus, as a student or practitioner of any particular theoretical medical philosophy, one's choice of action is controlled by the prevailing available solutions, theories and procedural policy of that system.

Following the above logic, it was clear to me that, even though these were women "seeing to this delivery," their actions were nevertheless controlled by the same frail human motivations that determine treatment, as well as administrative policy. To me, it boiled down to amount of empathy and degree of efficacy. Maybe this treatment was not as bad as that employed, whereby the "delivering mother" is strapped up in the air like a mule (This method of delivery, according to Mendelsohn, became official medical procedure due to the influence of King Luis XIV, whose perverted desire to watch women's vaginas was best satiated by such an angle of delivery. This awkward birthing position had nothing to do with any medical consideration, in fact, it actually causes baby to have to fight gravity to get into this world.). And, maybe she was not cruelly mishandled—as she was in her first pregnancy, whereby, according to "her say," a tall, masculine looking, hard faced, pale, dark haired white woman, who had compassion for no one, regardless of color, as she yelled: "You wudn't screaming when you opened up yo legs and got dat young'un, so shet up and open yo legs wida." Nevertheless, she (my wife) must have felt humiliation, and consternation from unfeeling, disdainful, and cold treatment that belied the claim of natural birth or Natural Birthing Room.

Accepting my role as "sensitive male protectorate," I monitored the variables that affect Mamaku's ability to carry out her birthing functions. I prayed that I could protect her from being hurt, which I had failed to do for my mother, even though my father had charged me with this duty in 1975, when he realized that he was dying from cancer (This is when I began studying Allopathic and Naturopathic methodologies, for my own understanding and peace of mind.)

My contemplations were interrupted, when our good friend the Lady Doctor came into the room. Boy, were we glad to see her. "She was all smiles," and with her greater authority, she was able to persuade those two nurses to "mind their manners." However, bless her heart, being trained and conditioned by Allopathic theory, practice and principle, she did the unthinkable-the very thing that made me convince my wife to stop using the women's clinic. After giving my wife a "passing grade," while turning to leave for her "appointed rounds," she swiftly reached her rubber glove clad fingers into that sacred place, that "hole-ly' place that I am sometimes still shy about reaching into (I feel this way, even when my wife coaxes me to use my fingers as a measuring device, in the name of that great "centimeter dilation hype," which you remember we disregard in favor of waiting on God and the baby), and she (the doctor) burst the amniotic sack. Doing so, she declared: "We'll just hurry things along a little, by breaking your water bag."

When she left. I became even more immobile, frozen in a catatonic state. Though my body was immobilized, the "OH MY GOD" thought, in my disbelieving mind, astonishingly enough, registered in the expression on my wife's face. My "Ghetto Paronoia" really took over then. "C-Section" loomed heavily on the horizon of my imagination.

Judging by the comments made by the two nurses, the possibility of C-Section as an option of delivery was not just my imagination. As they performed their mechanical tasks without warmth or compassion, they spoke loud enough for us to hear. Speaking as if C-Section was on their minds too, they seemed to deliberately make us privy to what they said to one another. They mentioned something about the baby's heartbeat, and they apparently felt as if Mamaku should by farther along . . . and that, no further dilation was evident.

Besides alarming me, and putting me on guard, this last comment was a profound testimony exposing the injurious nature of that little "hurry-up-bag-breaking-procedure." (My wife confirmed my suspicions about this procedure, some time later. She informed me that, at the very instant her friend broke her water bag, she realized that she was in danger, because immediately she felt a ceasation of the waves of contractions, which had begun to grow in intensity. In an attempt to get me to appreciate what that felt like, she described a similar sensation, to which I could relate. She said, instead of a mounting crest of waves, she felt a let down akin to the one that comes when someone walks into the bathroom while you are attempting a bowel movement. The "movement" retracts (like the baby), and there is a long wait before the urge gets under way again. She also reported that, at that very instant, she instinctively knew that she had to take steps to prevent the dreaded "intervention fruit operation"-C-Section. She said that she closed her eyes-which I noticed at the time-and, went deep within herself. She stated that she visualized herself traveling back deep into the Nile Valley, where she allowed the clear blue waters of the Nile River to flow through her body. She prayed that this action would give our baby an encouraging and gentle ride "home." She prayed to Imhotep, to Aton Ra, to Allah and Jah, to God and to Jesus. She said she prayed to all our Gods for help, to bring our baby forth.)

Miraculously enough, the moment our Doctor friend returned, Mamaku, displaying all the bravery of a true modern heroine, "squeezed" the baby's wrinkled crown into view. Moments later, the baby-who we would name Rahkua-popped her little head out. However, when her head pushed up to the neck, a sobering gush of blood sprayed out like a red hula skirt fountain. Her head was framed by blood shooting out all around. Her eyes, nose and mouth-before it opened to release a "milk-curdling scream"-were outlined by the color of red blood.

She was a nervous wreck! Both Mother and Child exhibited an uncontrollable nervous tremble, and involuntary shudder. (Rahkua's tremble lasted for several months; it would resurface regularly, until it finally wore off, perhaps because of a steady addition of Catnip, and Chickweed herb tea to her diet of Mother's milk.)

Natural Birthing Wing indeed; what a joke! We can laugh now, but it wasn't so funny then. I can't for the life of me imagine how they could figure that there was anything natural about that room, or what went on in it. We are natural people, by virtue of the laws of nature we recognize, and God's law, to which our freed souls submit. We were misled into believing that our beliefs, and naturopathic practices would be accommodated. They were not. We were not allowed to use our natural remedies, and when we declared that we did not approve of the "black gook" and electrical monitoring devices put on Mamaku's belly, and the unnatural silver nitrate being put into our baby's eyes, we were rudely overruled. They dumped that silver nitrate into Rahkua's eyes against our wishes. They even ignored our instructions concerning our intentions for Rahkua to be breast-fed. A "seemingly" sweeter nurse, who had returned with our Doctor friend, shoved a bottle of "formula" into Rahkua's mouth, blatantly disregarding our wishes. And, those other nurses, well let's just say that they were no Florence Nightingale, nor did they possess the warm healing qualities like the ones possessed by the nurses who saved Robert J. Ringer's wife.

In short, neither that Natural Birthing Wing, nor the administrators responsible for running it, reflected an understanding of anything remotely resembling natural child-birth. That natural birth room experience did, however, serve my cause well, though, because Rahkua did receive the gift of life there, and just as importantly, from that point forward, I had no more problems convincing Mamaku that our interests and beliefs would best be served, if we conducted our own births at home (which would turn out to be four more)!

Anyway, what were we talking about?. Oh yeah, the birthing room environment.

While we continue our discussion of the important role that the birthing room environment plays in the birth process, I must inform my reader of what is happening as we write.

It is ten minutes to 1:00AM, Friday Night (if you will), Nov. 2nd, 1996. I am tired; I've been working on my roof all day. It's cold, and I am "smack dab" in the middle of replacing five ceiling joists. I am doing this major project by myself, and there is quite a bit of work left. I've got to jack up the roofing joists, and replace 5, which were rotted, and tie them into the sills-which I had to replace. Then, I'll be able to replace the gaping hole in the roof, which was directly above our bedroom. After that I have to cover the hole, and the joists with plywood, before covering that with felt paper, roofing cement, and desert sand colored roll roofing.

Everyone else is asleep. I am writing, and thinking of the conversation I had with my wife before she fell asleep on the "pallet" in front of our Gallery fireplace. I know I promised not to tell any more stories, but at this very moment, I am hoping that my wife will add the story of our Grand son's birth, to this manuscript. This story, also unfolded in a local hospital. When I read the last story about Rahkua's birth, to my wife, the mention of C-Section jogged her memory of Jaylon's birth. Our discussion about these stories is very significant, in that, the brainstorming we did, while comparing notes about possible causes of this terrible complication, led us to make an earthshaking conclusion about this medical procedure.

If my wife blesses our literary efforts with her wonderful writing style Tomorrow, I'll include it after the summary discussion on birthing room environment.

Well, it is two days later, Sunday afternoon, Nov. 3rd, 1996, and Mamaku is reading, "Song Of TheTrees," by Mildred Taylor. The whole family is sitting, well, . . . the boys are jumping around, and trying to listen between giggles. I'm writing, and facing the fact that I can forget about relying on Mamaku to write that story about our Grandson's "near" C-Section birth. The urgent need to complete this manuscript, won't allow me to wait any longer. I guess this "is" a book written from the man's perspective, so I'll just finish without her written in-put. However, the reason that I wanted to include that story revolves around an alarming statistic that Mendelsohn reveals in "Male Practice." He approximates that 80% of the babies that are born by C-Section, are done so unjustifiably. It occurred to me, that the need for this "drastic, belly cutting method of delivery," is created by the frivolous use of that little innocent looking "bag breaking procedure" we just discussed in our last story.

The story that Mamaku told me about our oldest daughter's delivery experience confirmed my theory of cause and effect, relative to C-Section response to delivery problems, which are actually caused by "bag breaking interference." I must tell this story myself, because the conclusions are significant, and may spark legitimate need for review and elimination of this harmful procedure.

When Mamaku revealed the story to me, I took particular notice of the fact that both she, and our daughter had the same reaction to **the "bag breaking procedure." In both cases, the baby's progress was impeded when the water bag was broken**. In turn, this "stalling" justified "Code Blue" alarm, signaling the need for surgical intervention, which immediately followed the unnatural breakage of the water bag.

According to Mamaku, even after she advised the "Head" Doctor that she did not want him to break our daughter's water bag, he did so anyway. "Oh Lord, what did he want to do that for!" He caught a glimpse of "Ninja Mama," when he tried to explain to her, "all authoritatively," that dilation had stopped increasing, and had actually begun to regress. He could scarcely conclude his prognosis, that the baby had gone back up, before Mamaku cut him off, screaming: "The baby did what?! . . . she was nine centimeters, only one centimeter away from delivery readiness!" Mamaku said she started "losing it," as she continued yelling. "Naw Mother fucker . . . , you done fucked up. You broke that water bag, and now you tryin' to justify cuttin' on my baby."

Then, according to Mamaku, she went to that "other place," as she added: "I know you tryin' to kill my baby. Well, I shook yo funky hands, not because

I wanted to greet you, but because I wanted to feel all inside you, and get in touch with your spirit. So, let me tell you something; if anything happens to my Daughter or my unborn Grandbaby, the first thing that is going to happen to you is that your little red "peeter" will turn black, shrivel up even smaller than it is, and fall off like dust, in yo nasty draws!"

Then, she said she turned, and stormed off, yelling and screaming into the nurses station, the following words-which were received by eyes that were glued to the floor: "You'd better take a good look at that Mother Fucker, 'cause that may be the last time you see him looking like that. 'Cause I'm gonna put the "Whomucktadoo" on his ugly ass!"

We'll end this last story by letting our reader know that Mamaku ran through the hospital screaming "Murderers in the house," along with a host of other choice "deliriums," as the "Head" doctor-who had brought in a colleague to support his somber official proclamation-excused himself, to go look at some charts. He did not return until after the nurse-whom he blamed for the baby's retreat into the womb-managed to get the situation under control. She coached our oldest daughter until dilation was once again wide enough, and she coaxed the baby until the top of his head brought sighs of relief.

That resourceful and understanding nurse pulled this delivery off by using techniques that my wife claims she has never before witnessed. She said that the nurse rushed over and peeped out of the door before closing it. Then, as she eyed the door, she gave our daughter instructions designed to bring her baby back down, conditioning her mind to make her body function properly. Instead of having daughter to lie on her side, in that original position-which seemed like an impossible delivery position in the first place, she instructed daughter to turn over on her back, and reach her arms and hands through, and around her thighs to grip each ankle, in sort of a rocking chair position. Then she told daughter to bear down as hard as she could, as if forcing out bowel.

The last word on that story is that, the nurse's method worked; our grandson came out just fine, thank you! . . . , and **he didn't need A, B, or C-Section . . .** , just a focused Mom, competent guidance, and assistance waiting on God. (We thank that beautiful nurse who showed our daughter love and compassion, and shared some "natural" medical wisdom and knowledge with us, for which we pray that "trouble doesn't come around her door," and she is eternally blessed.)

This story affirms my faith that God controls natural birth, and if we love our mate, we will make sure that she gets safe treatment, devoid of procedures that interfere with the natural birthing process, especially when interference leads to problems that justify harmful and extreme medical intervention.

Furthermore, as I mentioned earlier, analysis of the significant points covered by the events of this story lead me to believe that we have unwittingly stumbled upon the reason for the high incidence of C-Section births: "premature doctor caused bag breaking." At any rate, with so much at stake, further research in this area is certainly warranted. Additionally, for me, any further use of this procedure raises moral, ethical, medical and legal questions.

To answer some of the questions surrounding the consequences of an inappropriate delivery technique that ends in artificial birth, deeply scarring the mother, and limiting her procreative functions perhaps permanently, we finish this episode by noting a few "educated" guesses and substantiated theories concerning C-Section birth. Then, before we continue our conclusion concerning the importance of delivery room environment, we make observations about the progress of our home birthing adventure book thus far.

First, though we admittedly base our conclusions on limited data deemed from our personal experience, nevertheless, we feel that perhaps Dr. Mendelsohn was off the mark by nearly 20%, when he proclaimed that 80% of C-Section births were unjustifiable. This means that said method of delivery is indefensible and needs to be discarded. (I know that some will disagree, and argue that this hypothesis and conclusion have not been scientifically verified. They may add that we do not have enough data from "controlled sampling," and random testing, etc. etc. However, as an honor student of political science, familiar with correlations, and projections and data manipulation, I am confident that we are "batting 1,000%, and our analysis is conclusively significant.)

If you want to talk about unscientific, what about the reasons that Doctors give to justify breaking a pregnant woman's water bag? These reasons appear to be quite frivolous, and unfeeling, not to mention the fact that they don't have any basis in medical need or scientific rationale. Here are the reasons we were given by the Doctors we consulted regarding the use of these ill-fated practices:

1 "It is done to check the water to see if it is clear, or shows signs of Meningitis."
2 "Its just a little step used to hurry contractions along."
3 "It's used to hasten the delivery."

As the high probability of C-Section seems to me to be a graver consequence than the possibility of problems that may result from ignoring use of this bag-breaking technique because of any of the above reasons, the employment of such avoidable intervention amounts to a frightening usurpation of authority, and a negligent use of power. It is scary to think that a woman's ability to reproduce a future generation of children can be so callously treated, and she can be so coldly handicapped.

Throughout our discussions of such medical treatments, including my wife's birthing experiences at home and beyond, we have exposed much about her inner make up. This exposure is the very point upon which we mentioned that we would end our observations. It is not absolutely necessary for me to include this "tidbit," but I'm in a "talkative" mood, so, please indulge me. What is it, you say? Well, it is about Mamaku's reluctance, and lack of enthusiasm about this book-which deals with our adventures in home birthing. She feels that I may be exposing too much of her personal life, and, in a "not too flattering light." Hopefully, this last conversation allayed her concerns. I let her know that my "intestinal reaction" leads me to believe that, since these stories are truthful and real (with very little embellishment), people who read them will respond in a "cool" and intelligent manner. They will realize that we all are psychological complexities, sweet and nasty, calm and excitable, smart and dumb, at different points in time. I further pleaded my case by convincing her that it is logical to conclude that it is unrealistic to only show the reader an image of that "sweet angelic side" of her (the one she used to sweep me off my feet). She seemed to "buy" that last "rap," and accept this graphic destiny, and is more at ease with this undeniable mission.

With all that out of the way, we can get back to our summary of our childbirth techniques.

Accordingly, I am now, more convinced than ever, that it is absolutely essential for the birthing room to be filled with love, and harmony, and a unified intent. Disharmony, discord, and methodological disagreement may lead to problems, and unnecessary obstacles for Mom and Babe, no matter where the birth occurs. The people, the spirit, and the atmosphere in the birthing room must be loving, warm, healing, and reverent, to ensure the best results for a natural outcome. This brings to mind the place, nature, and circumstances surrounding the birth of Jesus. If you look at his birth from the perspective of whether or not it happened according to the kind of conditions that we believe are the most conducive for a safe and divinely sanctioned situation, it appears that he was born in the most natural of conditions possible. He was surrounded by his Mother, his Earthly and Heavenly Father, agreeable spirits, and loving creatures. No one attempted to intervene in that process. There were no Drugs, no electrical monitoring devices, no stirrups, no surgical incisions, nor anxious fingers to hasten or impede that glorious birth. (And we say we want to be more like Jesus.!)

At ant rate, once the proper environment is established, and the expectant Mom is monitored with the understanding that the baby is "on God's time," then the proper attitude is in control of the situation, and the correct "vibe" permeates the natural home birth circumstance. This protects the birth from the consequences of unwarranted intervention, and procedures that are not based on medical, spiritual, or scientific considerations.

Once the above conditions are met, including those mentioned in Chapters 1 and 2, the Expectant Dad is ready to assist his baby up, and out of that sweet love canal.

As an Expectant Dad, my assistance in the birthing act has included, "rapping" to Mamaku, filling her head with soothing words of encouragement, and praise. While speaking these words, and often praying with her, I also give her a gentle massage, concentrating on her belly, and the "taint," to promote elasticity, and ensure that it doesn't tear.

When the baby starts coming, after all the panting and coaxing and crying out, with a poker face, this "Mid-husband" must control his fears, overcome obstacles, and provide solutions for any complication that may arise. After helping the baby out, Mom's thigh seems to be the best place for him/her to rest for a moment. Then, the cord has to be clamped in two places, an inch apart and an inch from the baby's belly. After the cord is cut, the baby has to undergo an over-all check, before he is cleaned and handed over to Mom. Then, Dad lets out a sigh of relief, while preparing and serving herb tea.

After the baby gets weighed, during the wait for the placenta to deliver, "messes" have to be cleaned up, and order has to be restored. Once the placenta delivers, it is buried in the back yard. (According to West African birth stories, two weeks after the placenta is buried, it is dug up, boiled, eaten, and drank.) Well, this Dad was unable to keep the boiling, and eating, and drinking part of this birthing tradition. The funny thing is that, as I fought with the idea of being a "He-man," and possibly reaping untold spiritual, and health benefits, our dog "Muru" got wind of my dilemma. She saved me from forever feeling guilty about not possessing the strength to follow tradition. Muru ate the whole thing! While I had been procrastinating, Muru dug three feet down, and uncovered the placenta feast wrapped in layers of plastic, inside of several plastic bags. I was actually relieved that the placenta was gone, even though I was still curious and intrigued by the idea of dining on it.

Anyway, let's get to the point. Once we have a successful birthing behind us, we consult professional medical help, for an examination of the baby. Now, Dad is ready for hours of interrupted sleep, with crying baby and a "calling" needy mother, both of whom are happy to return the loving attention.

That concludes our overview of our birth experiences, and prepares us for our final analysis, and synthesis of the ideas, facts, experiences, and theories we covered in our exposure of the Ishakarah Family's Home Birthing Adventures.

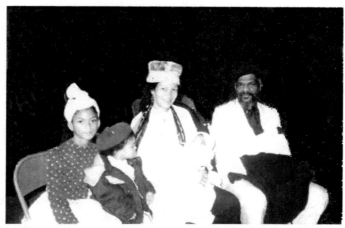

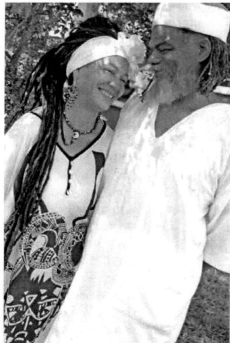

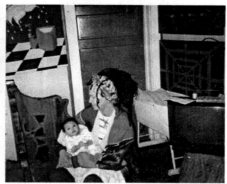

Top: photo of 5th daughter Rahkua, 6th daughter Namibiyah, and Mama Akua holding baby Rahzizi at a Davis Magnet School Christmas program in 1997 photo by Daisy Garrett digitally enhanced by RahLeeCoh

Left: Mama Akua and Baba RahLeeCoh share happy times in 2009; photo by Monica Holder

Right: Mama Akua holding Namibiyah surrounded by RahLeeCoh's Art

CHAPTER 7

CONCLUSION

This is our final chapter. Hoorah, we're nearly ready for the Oprah Show . . . well, our dream is to be her guest discussing this book!

In this chapter we make some far-reaching judgements, and show correlations between negative evolutionary trends and the loss of traditional values, particularly those related to a "fruitful" approach to family planning and growth. We also extol the virtues of our method of home birthing, as well as our life style choices. We philosophize about our "New Age" approach to seeking a modern lifestyle, which takes advantage of some traditional values that still have merit. This includes looking at the theoretical justifications for adopting a holistic approach to "Seeding and Harvesting" human life. (please excuse me for inserting this last analogy. I couldn't resist it. This appropriate phrase we lift from Rev.Creflo Dollar's sermon of yesterday, Sunday, October 27, 1996. His timely message was so eloquent, and profoundly related to the Ishakarah Family's own procreative ideology. The axiom that connects the point of Rev. Dollar's message to our home birthing philosophy is: "Positive actions nurtured, yield desired fruitful rewards.") Thank you Rev. Dollar. It is true that after a "youthhood" of celibacy, and an adulthood of strong divine communion, along with a quest for health consciousness, God blesses me and my wife with parenthood at a time when people our age (50 and 43 respectively) are contemplating retirement. As a result, we are now harvesting a youthful mind, a viable body, and beautiful little children. By putting our beliefs into practice, we have made ourselves available to receive God's rewards regarding the knowledge, will and ability, and health needed to manage our own "human fruit harvest."

A fitting close to this book of the Ishakarah family's adventures in home birthing must begin with contemplation on Mamaku's alleged miscarriage. This mishap represents the only strike against our home birth methods. Even though Blue convinced us that this "stuff" happens all the time, even in the hospital, we are still left with some questions, like: "Where did she begin? When was she conceived? Did we violate a natural law, or commit a sin? What must we do to avoid such a consequence in the future? Did we (I) rush into sex too soon? Did we do it any differently? To these questions, I can honestly answer: I don't know. I don't know. I don't know. And, I don't

96

think so. I don't think we "did it" anymore than we have in the past. Yet, maybe Ra Un Nefer Amien was correct when he proclaimed that too much copulation could be harmful. The thought occurs to me: "What about our Grandparents, and our Great Grandparents, were they wrong to give birth to so many children (16 or 20 children was not uncommon, yet today that fruitful two parent headed family has become small fragmented single parent households)?

Our "fore-parents" of the Twenties and Thirties definitely fulfilled scripture, to a greater extent than we do today. They were more fruitful, and they multiplied more than we do. Did they "do it" too much? May be not.

In fact, I think we may have been sold a "Bill of no good," in the sixties and seventies, when we eagerly absorbed "so called" middle class values, and a materialistic morality. We were taught to strive for a six-figure bank account, a two-car garage, and 1.5 children. This emphasis on material consumption and the accumulation of wealth, at the expense of spiritual growth and recognition of spirituality as an essential aspect of life," was the "pillow" of the "American Dream."

Here in Mississippi, even with its reputation for past racial atrocities, when the families were larger, it seems that we were closer, and people were warmer and more loving. Everybody waved (all races), and spoke when they passed. During those times, you could leave your house for weeks at a time, with your door open. You would return to find a bushel of corn, or sweet potatoes waiting inside your screen door. I can still remember the kind of Mississippi described by Dr.King. Grandma's house was a prime example of this "down home," country farm life style, governed by Christian Doctrine, and led by Grandpa's pure evangelical love ministry, back in those woods of Prentiss, Mississippi.

During those times, and even in the generation to follow, not only were babies born at home, but, people "made time" for one another, and "looked after" their loved ones. For the most part, our elderly, and our infants were taken care of at home, and they played an important part in the running of the household (even the elderly played a role in the running of the household). People had more respect, and more love for one another, and a greater sense of responsibility for the well being of neighbors and relatives; WE NEED THAT KIND OF CARING NOW!.

Today's generation is born in the hospital, and by an alarming percent of "birth by cutting" the mother open. These babies are then fed and nourished with bottle formulas, and cow's milk. The bonding and "humanizing" nature of the "act of nursing"(which connects the infant to mother's warmth, and allows for healing and the protection against diseases that is afforded by Mother's milk) has all but been eliminated. Breast feeding is almost seen as vulgar, and even criminal. As a result, in my opinion, we are more distant, and nearly numb to the feelings of others. We put our old parents in homes, and our children into Day Care facilities. We practice individualistic philosophies, and are versed only in one career profession. We have become profit motivated, at the expense of equity and justice. In short, we have become a society of less caring, and cold citizenry (unless there is a natural disaster, which usually brings humanity out of us).

I see a direct relationship between the loss of those traditional values just mentioned, adoption of the above modes of living, and evolvement to "drive by shooting," "freeway robbery," "exploding spark plug windshield highway assaults," "car jacking," "pipe bombings," horrible heinous murders, and other such acts of violence. Other problems seem to be attributable to this imbalance caused by material preoccupation. There is no question that our youth of today see "gangster rap," with its shameless callous language, as an acceptable and viable means of achieving financial materialistic success-a way of escaping the impoverished nightmares of a disenfranchised American. (This is the epitome of a "Catch 22" situation, because though the language of most rap music may be considered vulgar or objectionable, it is clear that these young ghetto poets have elevated the art of lyrical rhyming to astronomical heights; each album contains enough literary genius to qualify for PHD level mastery.) These same youth, whose parents "spared the rod," and whose schools removed God, and corporal punishment from the classroom, have little respect for anyone, and they are quick to resolve disputes with fire arms (Can you remember when a good old fist fight used to resolve our differences? Well, I guess they weren't so good, and occasionally there was a razor or a knife used in the battle, but at least the combatants usually survived to become friends and get older.).

Anyway, the point is that, we have evolved to a culture of weaker, fast paced, tense, drug abusive, and elusion dependent citizens, in need of spiritual grounding, and physical and mental healing. We need role models living amongst the populace demonstrating alternative lifestyle choices and providing positive solutions to problems due to living circumstances (such role models as "Positive Evolutionary Healing Agents," "New World Health Aestheticians and Visionaries," and, "Righteousness and Salvation Practitioners."). Of course, supporting such normative and idealistic solutions to the negative consequences of human evolution, presupposes that we can and should change the evolvement of our attitudes and behavior, that there are choices available to affect a change in the course our society can take, and that the present course is undesirable, and will end in a catastrophe that can and should be avoided.

What can we do about this evolution that reveals a pattern of growing greedy behavior that forsakes even "blood," while feeding an insatiable materialistic gluttony? And, what about the corruption, and the violence, the callous unjust treatment, the human rights violation, and the growing lack of love and respect: what can we do about it? Should we try to do anything about it?

As an American citizen living under the influence of the above negative evolutionary factors, I see the need to keep certain traditional values alive. I see a direct relationship between a loss of viable healing forces, and the lack of widely supported and utilized natural and traditional medical systems. For me, the solution to these negative manifestations lies in reinstating such values and practices as birthing children at home, and caring for their health using such natural means as providing them with a diet comprised mainly of fresh field and garden food, and exposing them to a cosmology that balances material preoccupation with diverse spiritual awareness, and the importance of creativity and self reliance.

This is why I am willing, and thanks to the grace of God, able to help my wife give birth to our children at home. (Now that's what I call reaching back to carry on a tradition. Because, you guessed it, I was actually born at home myself, to two beautiful and loving souls-Joseph and Arvella Courts, on July 4th, 1946, at 719 W. Pascagoula Street, here in Jackson Mississippi.)

Yet, my own personal evolvement to believing in the merits of a natural approach to childbirth developed as a consequence of my decision to pursue my love for art creation, despite the fact that my collegiate plans and career goals were aimed at Federal Judgeship.

My life as a Creative Artist put me on a path that required a "working relationship with God." I received "Divinely Inspired Visions and Messages," which formed the basis for much of my art creation. I also received the will to study many disciplines and professional occupations. This quest was aided by the Graduate level analytical skills, and curriculum development abilities I acquired as a student of Political Science. As it turned out, I needed to be able to perform various professional functions to supplement my secluded life style, which I funded with grass roots level art production and sales. Thus, obtaining a fair degree of comfort and security in a society that measures worth in terms of material possessions put a lot of pressure on my spiritually oriented personality. That is why, living life as a so called "Starving Artist," meant that I had to constantly devise means and methods of generating enough capital to support an acceptable standard of living. This called for a high degree of self-sufficiency. Yet, such efforts only generated below poverty level income, which meant that I had to live on a budget that did not include expenses for hiring an Accountant, nor the services of an

Auto Mechanic, nor contracting with a Carpenter or Plumber, not to mention, the lack of funds needed to hire the counsel of an Attorney. Sometimes I could barter, let's say, a painting for some dental work. But, by and large, I've had to wear all the hats mentioned. (This does not include Accounting, my weakest subject in College. Hell, I couldn't understand that little foreign guy. Even if I could keep up with his words, I still couldn't translate them, so I dropped out of class.).

I attribute my ability and daring to study various disciplines, and employ them when needed, to the impression my father put on my mind, by way of the example of his industry. He demonstrated the model of a man who, with only a sixth grade education, succeeded in gaining knowledge and skills enough to rebuild auto motive engines, repair household appliances and TV.'s and accomplish just about whatever he "set his mind to." This included providing a working class living, as a baker with the A&P Bakery, for himself, his wife and five sons.

The need for self-sufficiency also led me to develop the ability to solve my own health problems. This could only be done after study, and use of Alternative Healing Arts Methods. I had to learn the principles of Holistic Health Care, and treat myself.

Acquiring expertise in the field of Alternative Medicine was a gradual learning and "unveiling" process. I can trace my resulting medical wisdom and acumen back to the inspiration provided by a University of Michigan coed, who gave me the gift of a "Tea¬Ball," for brewing herb tea, and a box of Red Zinger Herb Tea. This act of love, and unselfish sharing got me "off and running," and it opened up a whole new world for me. It was a world of Health Wizards (this is a different view of the intelligent people who are knowledgeable on the subject of health, instead of the demeaning stigma: health nut. Did I mention that there is nothing nutty about a person who is concerned about their health, and is willing to be "socially incorrect," or oppose popular opinion when it comes to choosing an effective method of staying well and fit.) It was a world of warm, health loving people of all kinds. Moreover, it was a world of Health Food Stores, and theories of dietary and "Herbological" treatment and cure for disease, of alternative health care philosophies, and principles of Mind/Body Healing for self and others.

I was awakened to a new reality, which drove me like an obsession, on a predestined path, gathering knowledge and understanding in the Healing Arts. I ate and drank health wisdom, synthesizing information, and comparing data from differing Alternative Healing Systems, while judging theoretical frameworks, and analyzing efficacy of treatment and level of cure. I arrived at conclusions about traditional and contemporary medical approaches, such as Naturopathy, Homeopathy, and Allopathy.

For me, raised with a strong Baptist grounding in the healing mission of Jesus, yet influenced by scientific methodology, the medical system I chose to use in my life had to account for the inseparable phenomenological nature of the human being. Directed by a "working" belief in the miracles possible through faith in God, the only possible choice of a health care system I could use had to operate on theory that recognized the unity of Mind/Body/Soul in its methods. The theory of that medical approach, had to demonstrate scientific principles that worked with and complimented the reality of a spiritual connection to the force and source of life—God.

Holistic Health Care Systems was the only choice I could make.

As I studied and practiced the methods of Herbology, Massage Therapy, Reflexology, and Vegetarianism, I began to discover overwhelming data proving that Alternative Healing Systems have a record of the most efficacious methodology. The information I accumulated on these medical systems revealed a history of data and results that are more satisfactory, without the so-called "side effects." After becoming well versed in this area, I came to recognize and believe that naturopathic procedures work because they are grounded in the irrefutable relationship between God, Nature, and the inseparable aspects of human mental, physical and spiritual being, especially when it comes to the wellness process.

Armed with the above knowledge, and beliefs, I was able to do battle with my own personal illnesses, and diseases. I was also able to help a few friends and loved ones solve their own health problems as well. The wisdom and courage I gained as a result of these experiences gave me the confidence to attempt the feat of managing the birth of our children at home. It has also allowed my wife and me to use Naturopathic solutions to remedy health problems our children encounter in their growth and development,

This reminds me of the sermon I was called, and requested to bring to my family's church at that time-The Precious Stone Church, pastured by Rev. M. Hollowell. As Health Minister for the church, I responded by praying and meditating for the message to bring to our congregation. Rev. Hollowell recorded the divinely inspired words that flowed through me (my wife also participated during the delivery of the sermon, by demonstrating the healing techniques of Hara). The title given to that sermon was: "Healing: The Component of Religion That Requires Contact With God."

During the process of composing, and writing the subject matter of this healing message, we received the following revelation: "God has been taken out of healing, and healing has been taken out of religion." This accounts for contemporary medical failure when it comes to "curing" Chronic Degenerative Diseases. (The Allopathic emphasis seems to rely too heavily on "seen relationships" and scientific and mechanical reasoning, upon drugging, cutting and treating symptoms, rather than getting to the core of the problem and finding a solution to the stress and strain caused by a fast paced modern style of living. Glory is given to scientific and technical means of treatment rather than the effective nature of the cure. In fact, we have all heard statements like, "she' s got a fifty/fifty chance, if we operate, but we can't guarantee anything," or "this treatment is just a means of keeping her comfortable as she dies.") Dr.Mendelsohn concurs with this revelation, when he intimates that the hospitalization process and routine has really become religious ritual, whereby, belief in God has been substituted with faith in the demeanor and rhetoric of contemporary doctors. This trust is so powerful that it influenced too many of my loved ones into submitting to insane operations that actually appeared to accelerate the death process, rather than bring about a healing cure. Faith in these doctors persuaded these same loved ones to ignore my pleas, and disregard research data revealing unbelievable failure rates for the operations that ended in horrible death. (Add my brother Sam to that list. After thirty days of radiation treatment "they" turned him, at 49 years old, into an eighty year old looking, black leathery skinned, "Tales Of The Crypt" like being, that my children didn't recognize, and that made my wife have to run to his bathroom to hide her tears, the last time we saw him. He was the closest person in my family to me, beside my Mother, yet, the "health nut" stigma prevented him from accepting my healing knowledge and assistance, and he rejected the research my wife and I did, and the Naturopathic program of cure we devised on his behalf. We miss him dearly because he was a true uncle to our children, and the only man in town, with whom we felt safe and secure about trusting around our daughters.)

This is why we were ready to bring God back into the birthing methods we developed from all the information we learned while seeking birthing know how. We believe so strongly in this position that we include the contents of the sermon we just spoke of, which reveals the path we've followed to arrive at our belief in God as the ultimate power source controlling the natural birth process. (See Appendix C) (I could tell you a good and juicy story about the events leading up to that blessed day, when we delivered the message. It would include how my family met Baba O.K, of "Arrest and Develop;" and how he added a special spiritual touch, as he attended that service and "Blessed the occasion," "Paying Homage to our Ancestors," by "Pouring Libations." But, I promised, no more stories, so, I won't. Maybe I'll include it in my next book!)

Taking our lead from the main premise of that sermon," Healing: The Component of Religion That Requires Contact with God," we recognize a "curative void" left in any practice of medicine that eliminates God from the solutions chosen to handle today's health problems. These Chronic Degenerative Diseases are the result of pressure filled life styles, driven by a desire to accumulate wealth, and founded on values upholding material acquisition and "Madison Avenue boosted Sex out of context." These modern illnesses germinate from a complex combination of factors, including poor eating habits, sedentary living, drug and alcohol abuse, and stress filled choices of action. The healing methods with the most viable and effective approach to these health problems submit to natural law. They provide solutions that deal with the wholeness of human being-which cannot be isolated, and separated. The treatments promoted by contemporary medical reasoning, appear to be founded on assumptions that view body parts as entities that can be separated out and treated to bring about a change for the better. My research and experiences prove this assumption to be false, which underscores the need to bring God back to the healing process, the sick bed, and especially, the birthing room.

For me, the above observation and conclusion are revelation; it implies correctness in the theory and practice of a Holistic Health Care System. It is the wisdom that leads to making the right decision, and taking the correct course of action. It puts our evolutionary trends into perspective, and it is proof that, in order for us to stem the tide of a Nation, "hell bent" on self destruction-characterized by mal-alligned individuals, capable of senseless and indiscriminant killing, while being directed by greed, we may have to re-evaluate our priorities. We may need to re-examine our emphasis upon so called Technological Advancements in medicine, and its connection to the profit motive. It may be necessary for us to develop new value systems, and styles of living that rename appropriate norms of behavior adapted to models created in anticipation of 21st Century problem solving.

Our final, and concluding contention is that such life style synthesis of the old, the contemporary, and the "yet uncreated," forms the basis for our personal evolvement to the point of wanting to have a lot of children, and to take responsibility for their birth, health, and guidance at home. We further sincerely believe that other parents with similar spiritual convictions, tenacious drive, and dedication to learning, and mastering the birthing process, with faith in God, can have success. They too can achieve the worthwhile goal of having their children at home, ensuring a more economical alternative. These parents may find, as we did, that home birth is the healthiest and safest way to go, with the proper safeguards and precautions. They may realize an additional benefit, in the form of a relationship affected positively by the leadership role that the "Proud Papa" must take. Assuming this responsibility will sensitize him to his wife's needs, and give him greater understanding of, and more empathy for her feelings and sufferings. This may lead to a closer family, comprised of happy parents, with a host of "remarkably gifted" and talented children, who radiate with beautiful, healing and loving smiles, like the ones our children have . . . OH THANK YOU GOD!

EPILOGUE

We ended our Conclusion by thanking God for all the wisdom, knowledge, and birthing experiences that allowed us to contribute a "how to" book to the world of literature. Yet, even though we also thanked God for our beautiful children, we were still disappointed by the fact that a possible miscarriage stood in the way of a perfect record of our birth management experiences. However, "Hallelujah," as we pull this literary effort closer to publication, we are glad to "bear witness to God's blessings, and merciful goodness." We have been allowed to redeem our failed attempt to collect scientific data on a birth process in progress. Though we discontinued our record keeping, Mamaku did become pregnant again, and we were blessed with another son, on the 30th day of November 1997.

To reward our faith and conviction regarding our home birth advocacy, Rahzizi-Sam-Q-Ademolahjah-E.J.-Verderosa-Ishakarah is "God's gift to bring (us) wealth, and settle disputes." He came to us after our miscarriage mishap, and his birth allows us to end this book on a positive note. Once again, we are confident about the techniques we use, and we are certain that these methods demonstrate quite clearly, "How we make babies, and give birth to them at home."

The story of Rahzizi's birth confirms the fact that my wife and I have "got this home birthing thing down pat." It has become second nature now, which is proven by the fact that we can improvise, and "make do," with what God provides us. In this case, we were the least prepared. Yet, at the last minute, we sterilized my old exacto knife blade, and a pair of unused shoestrings, and guided Rahzizi safely into this world, as, for the first time, his siblings watched in amazement. This success, thanks to God, assures us that we were correct in our assessment that views the natural birth process as largely a spiritual phenomenon. It also affirms my contention that our method is scientifically sound, and deserves consideration for broad scale use by potential fathers and mothers who desire to give life to their children at home, and share this wonderful and rewarding adventure.

APPENDIX A

MAMA AKUA'S BIRTH

PROGRESS

CHART

DATE: June 12, 1996

DIET:

BREAKFAST: toasted French bread. Brown Rice Grits, soy margarine, honey, soy sausages, and herb water (made by dilluting a sauce pan of herb tea in a gallon of water)

LUNCH: "fake'n bake'n samidge" (soy bean/vegetable protein product), with lettuce and tomatoes, soy mayonnaise, mushroom tofu omelet on wheat toast, and lemon aide made with honey and bottled water

DINNER: brown rice, split peas and carrots, raisin com bread, and lemon aide made with honey and spring water

OBSERVATIONS:
Mamaku rested a great deal, complaining of a headache and neck ache; she had a voracious appetite, ate three helpings of dinner and made skillet bread snack later

REMEDIES AND SOLUTIONS:
Mamaku drank two large glasses of herb tea water (made with diluted solutions of peppermint and comfrey)
She received a neck massage; and, later, a total body massage with olive oil

ACTIVITIES:
She went for walks in the neighborhood; once in the morning with Rah-Imhotep, and later with the whole family

APPENDIX B

"SONG FOR TITUBA"

By: Akua Ishakarah

As a "Journalism Medium," 1 received the following words, and they flowed through me, in tribute to Margie Conde's great novel: "I Tituba, Black Witch Of Salem." We shall refer to my creative response to Conde's work as: "Song For Tituba" (Titled by my husband, RahLeeCoh Ishakarah). Conde's inspirational and creative ending to Tituba's life suggested the possibility of a spiritual rebirth to allow for a healing remedy to a tragic and horrible human injustice. This suggestion took root in my mind, and grew into a narrative revelation, which begins with the last two lines of Conde's courageous journalism: "I was the last to be taken to the gallows. All around me strange trees were bristling with strange fruit." (p.172)

The wind began to howl with such fury that Errin, and the rest of the "God fearing Planters" fell to their knees in unison. They began thrusting both hands forward, flailing them up and down, and, with heads lowered, started crying-begging for mercy, and shouting for Satan to let go of God's children.

At will, the howling subsided, allowing only an uncertain pause of deafening silence, before all eyes took notice of the dancing leaves. They were swaying to the rhythm of a soft, haunting whistle. The mesmerizing sound was caused by the wind's caress of each branch of those unforgiving trees-whose roots pounded, like ancient "down beats," echoing ancestral seeds.

The salty foam, now drying on the end of my tongue, ate away any possible sound. Even groans of agony were silenced. Now, that whole frothy white, pinkish appendage thickened like a big honey sweet, and juicy, sun ripened mango. The smile on my face reflected in the amazed, and fearful glances of guilt glued to the image of those standing before me. They were the true wicked ones in this horrible situation. They were consumed by horrified grimaces, as they consciously denied their guilt, while watching in disbelief, as Mama Yaya, Abena my mother, and Yao-my God given father-took me by the hands, and joined each other's hands. Hand in hand, they created a spiritual link between my physical body, and their invisible world. Then, after giving me an ancient and mystical glance, they seemed to become visible, as they turned slowly to face our persecutors. An incredible beam of red fury bolted from their melded, and penetrating eyes. That focused, and piercing ray appeared to have a single purging intent; it sought out Errin, and the others who had skillfully mastered the art of cruelly destroying our healers, and damning our concerned leaders. That light of justice closed in on these same evil masters who had showed no feelings as they used merciless whips, and brutal hangman's knots, tied so cleverly and applied so coldly.

The "avenging beam of justice" quickly sealed the fate of the pleading persecutors, as their unforgiven souls turned to unrecognizable heaps of ashes, and began to swirl. This powerful circular force moved amongst the rest of the evildoers-the bearers of false witness-churning like a tornado of hornets. With relentless stinging "blows," all those tainted souls were driven into the upset "Barbadoen" waters, where they were eagerly met by angry waves, crested from centuries of bloody tears and pain filled sweat. This precipitation resulting from tumultuous injustice, whose loins harvested pounding tides, left no trace or rememberance of the "real" practitioners of evil-those whose evil deeds had been hidden under the guise of "God fearing Masters," and innocent spectators out for an evening of "harmless" fun.

Their work done, as a holy trinity, Mama Yaya, Abena, my mother, and Yao, my God given father, embraced me, freed me, and carried me on a transcendental voyage to Paradise.

My glorious healing gave birth to a beautiful girl child-Rahealyah. A faint blue halo, graced by a pinkish hue-not quite visible, adorned her head; humbly illuminating her sand tented Dread Locks. Rahealyah, empowered with the touch of miracles, which flow throughout the purity of her corpuscles, gives health filled life to those who are worthy. Those so blessed to behold her beauty and embrace her healing love are rewarded with the happiness of healthy living, as a way of life which showers our universe with Utopian soil.

Now, my work is also done, fulfilled by Rahealyah's vindicating mission, I can rest In peace.

Amen-Rah

APPENDIX C

Healing: The Component Of Religion

That

Requires Contact With God

Sermon by: RahLeeCoh Ishakarah
(Precious Stones Church
Minister Of Health)

I. INTRODUCTION

"How strong is your faith? (Mathew 8:13)

A strong faith in God, and love in your heart, allows healing to occur. So, why is it that we submit to operations, and a practice in general, that are neither spiritual, nor "in keeping" with the laws of nature, violate healing principles, and ignore the healing methods employed by Jesus?

Today, our God has been taken out of the healing process, so that now, the part of religion practiced by Jesus, namely healing the mind and the body using a variety of methods, has been removed from religious practice. That process has now become scientific, and secular procedure, and evolved to the point of becoming medical decisions, and actions based on the erroneous assumption that scientific methodology is superior, and more effective than faith in God. This has made it easy for people to delude themselves into believing that it is possible to sin all week, and yet, be saved by going to Church on Sunday. This allows for suffering under the delusion that a sinful secular life can exist along side, and yet, be separated from such a psuedo-religious one. Thus, our minds are conditioned to believe, and socialized to think that "cures" for illnesses are quick, and simple. This same logic, which automatically follows a system of "sinning all week and absolution on Sunday," persuades us into believing that, since the medical solutions are quick and simple, we can get back to doing the same self-destructive kinds of things that caused the medical and health problems in the first place. However much we pretend

110

that these modern methods are more sophisticated and work, statistical data analysis demonstrates otherwise.

II. INEFFECTIVE NATURE OF CONTEMPORARY MEDICAL SOLUTIONS

A. Current health care crisis result of modern medical inability to provide methodological answer to questions about the spiritual portion of modern pathology

1 Toxic, poisonous, nutritionally deficient life styles, full of stressfilled bad habits, and self-destructive thinking patterns and behavioral responses to fast paced society, produce complex modern illnesses, sickness and disease

2 The prevailing, legally dominating medical system reports a documented history of data showing a record of treatment that fails to cure chronic degenerative diseases

3 Anyone desiring to be cured of such diseases, is obliged to challenge allegiance to inappropriate technology, and seek curative understanding provided by alternative medical systems with better records of cure, then make a comparative analysis of efficacy of allopathic methodology, as opposed to naturopathic means, before choosing the preferred treatment

B. Modern Medical Treatment and its Erroneous Underlying Assumptions Vs Ancient Healing Teachings and Traditional Medical Cures

1. Comparative look at the theoretical foundation of modern medicine

a. The fundamental error of western scientific medical theory occurs when it ignores the metaphysical, and spiritual realm of being, basing its conclusions on physical deductions that allow for fragmentation of the world, justifying a separation of religion from daily living, and separation of body parts and organ systems from the whole self (Ra Un Nefer Amein pp. 3,4, &6)

b. Wrongful viewpoint led the dominant medical system (AMA) into thinking that diseases are always "out there" in a continuous battle with the body

c. Proceeding as if the body is in a continual adversarial relationship with disease, and the body is a divisible entity, Western medical theory operates as if it can be separated from the mind, and the spirit, which is precisely the logic used to justify removal of organs and parts that are declared diseased beyond repair, however, doing so without first advising the patient that the rest of the body will be drained and weakened, and have to make up for the loss, which in some cases (like that of my own parents) is insurmountable, and death is accelerated, as inadequate interference fails miserably, causing toxins to spread rapidly, unchallenged by natural defenses, which are eliminated by this method of treatment

d. The treatment leading to the above "iatrogenic" nightmare is erroneously justified by mistaken modern medical theory and the presupposition that "drugging and cutting" can bring about a cure (though the "Allopaths" only claim to "treat") for our degenerating physical and mental condition, yet their very own data demonstrates just the opposite, which leads me to conclude that these actions are no less than criminal, especially since I received the word "GERONTICIDE," from my mother, as she communicated with me after her death, at the unmerciful hands of this modern medical system that "treated" her to a hole sawed into her skull for her loyalty and medicinal use of Dilantin prescribed for her degeneration (in effect, geronticide is a descriptive testimony to the elimination of the elderly using pharmaceutical addictive attrition, and surgical destruction)

2. Looking intelligently at the basic underlying principles of Alternative Health care systems available for the choosing (despite the negative press given to any selections outside of the mainstream bandwagon), for the purpose of selecting the best method for use on self and family, particularly the one which seems most sane, more humane, and yes even most important, more Godly, a reasonable person should conclude, and recognize the wisdom and effectiveness inherent in the Health Teachings of the Ancients, and the efficacious viability of traditional medical systems in general (Ra Un Nefer Amen pp.6-7)

a. the whole being is considered in any program of health care, and improvement (Holistic health care)

b. Nature's natural cures are incorporated into the therapy, Including sunshine, fresh air, pure water, herbs of the field, and exercise, along with plenty of rest and relaxation

c. Traditional Medical Systems also recognize the spiritual Essence of the human being, while seeking to attain divine influence in the healing process, allowing for reclamation of birth rites established by Aton, and Amon Ra, giving access to wellness through prayer, and healing directives not provided by the failed solutions of modern medical principles

III. JESUS' HEALING MISSION

Proof that healing is an indispensable part of religion rests in the example that Jesus provided in his works, which display several healing techniques that seem To be of the highest level possible within the art and science of healing; several of These methods are recorded in the King James Version of the Bible, particularly

In Matthew 4 :24;8: 15

A. Laying on of hands-{Matthew 8: 1-3) and (Mark 6 : 32-35)
B. Spoken Word-(Mark 6: 34)
C. Prayer/MeditationlFasting-(Matthew 4 : 2)
D. Spittal in the dust
E. Cleansing Leprosy, and Using Herbs

IV. BRIEF DESCRIPTION OF ALTERNATIVE HEALING SYSTEMS

The imperative challenge for those concerned about truly effective medical treatment, involves the need for comparative analysis and restoration of influence, understanding, and employment ofTraditional, and Holistic Medical Theory and Practice

A. Herbology   B. Vegetarianism   C. Macrobiotics
D. Massage   E. Yoga   F. Fasting   G. Meditation and Hara

V. CONCLUSION

Recognizing the fact that healing was a very important aspect of Jesus' Mission, makes it easy to understand that healing is definitely a religious activity. Understanding that contemporary medical science has been used to authorize, and legally protect a crafty take over of the right to choose a form of medical treatment that cooperates with natural human spirituality, leads to the conclusion that political intrigue was used to promote an officially sanctioned nature of cure, and consequently pervert the importance of natural healing, thus divesting it of meaning for the treatment and wellness process. This perversion includes the manner in which modern medical personnel, and the hospitalization system have joined forces (funded by insurance money, and protected by sympathetic laws and law makers) to create a system of medical treatment that has become a sort of religion in and of itself. Those who submit to such practices, unwarily give this modern system the power to replace God in the methods validated as legitimate means for curing their bodies (p.8 "Natural Healing Through Macrobiotics").

What can we do about getting our God back into the methods used for the purpose of healing our bodies? How can we put healing back into our religious beliefs and practices?

A. See the need for establishing a healing forum, study and practice component in our religious programs which become an integral part of our everyday life
B. We must bury our fears (evoking fear is the primary tactic used to condition our minds to accept indefensible operations), and anxieties in the exercise of our faith-a faith that recognizes God as the power behind all healing, and develop enough courage to face our health problems relying on divine guidance
C. We must develop our cognitive skills, intuitive logic, and analytical abilities, in order that we become able to make intelligent choices, as we rely on our own instincts and insights
D. We must be willing to change our bad habits, our negative actions, and our wrongful thoughts, and acknowledge the fact that the body in our "being" was not isolated when illness came about, and as such cure has to account for the total self, which includes a spiritual aspect that makes religion and God inseparable parts of the healing treatment in order for wellness to be a viable result

APPENDIX D

PRINCIPLES

OF

HEALTHY LIVING

GET PLENTY OF FRESH AIR, BREATH DEEPLY PERIODICALLY
DRINK FREELY OF PURE WATER
EAT ONLY OF NATURE'S FRESH FRUIT, VEGETABLES, NUTS, &
GRAIN
SUPPLEMENT THE DIET WITH VITAMINS AND MINERALS
"KNOW THE HERBS OF THE FIELD," & THEIR HEALING
PROPERTIES
EXERCISE REGULARLY, AND VIGOUSLY IN THE SUNSHINE
PRACTICE THE HEALING ARTS: YOGA, MASSAGE,
VEGETARIANISM
FAST, IMMEDIATE, AND PRAY FOR MIND/BODY STRENGTH
TAKE FREQUENT BATHS, AND CLEANSING ENEMAS
MAINTAIN LOVE, ORDER AND CLEANLINESS AROUND YOU
REFRAIN FROM DRUG USAGE AND DEPENDENCY
TAKE RESPONSIBILITY FOR YOUR OWN GOOD HEALTH

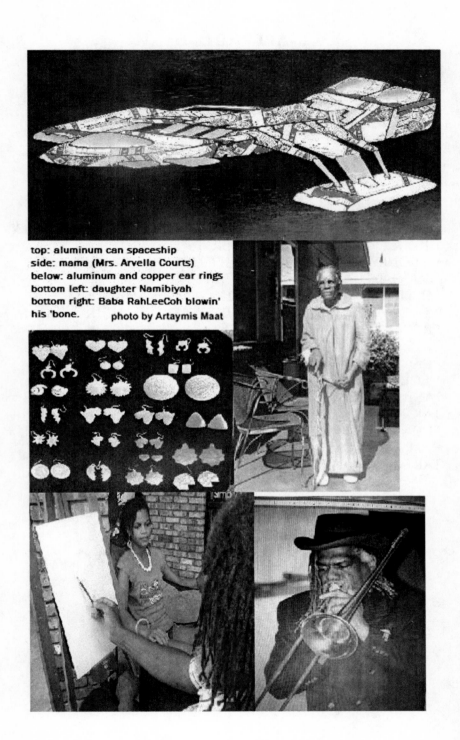

top: aluminum can spaceship
side: mama (Mrs. Arvella Courts)
below: aluminum and copper ear rings
bottom left: daughter Namibiyah
bottom right: Baba RahLeeCoh blowin'
his 'bone.   photo by Artaymis Maat

LaVergne, TN USA
23 December 2010

209941LV00004B/44/P